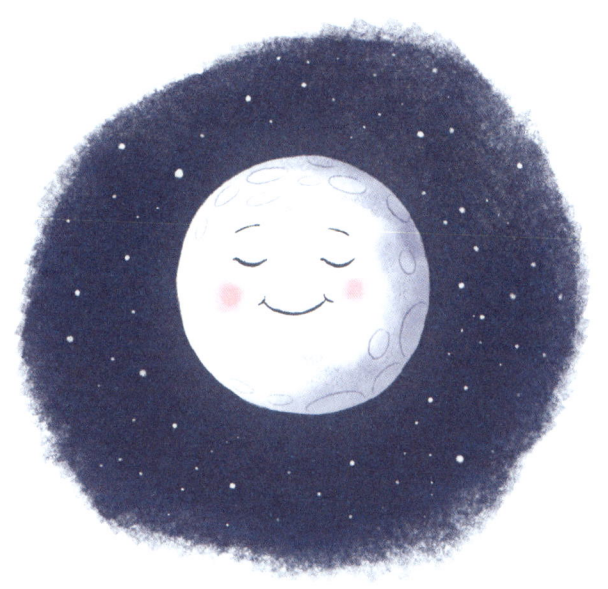

THE SLEEP SCAN

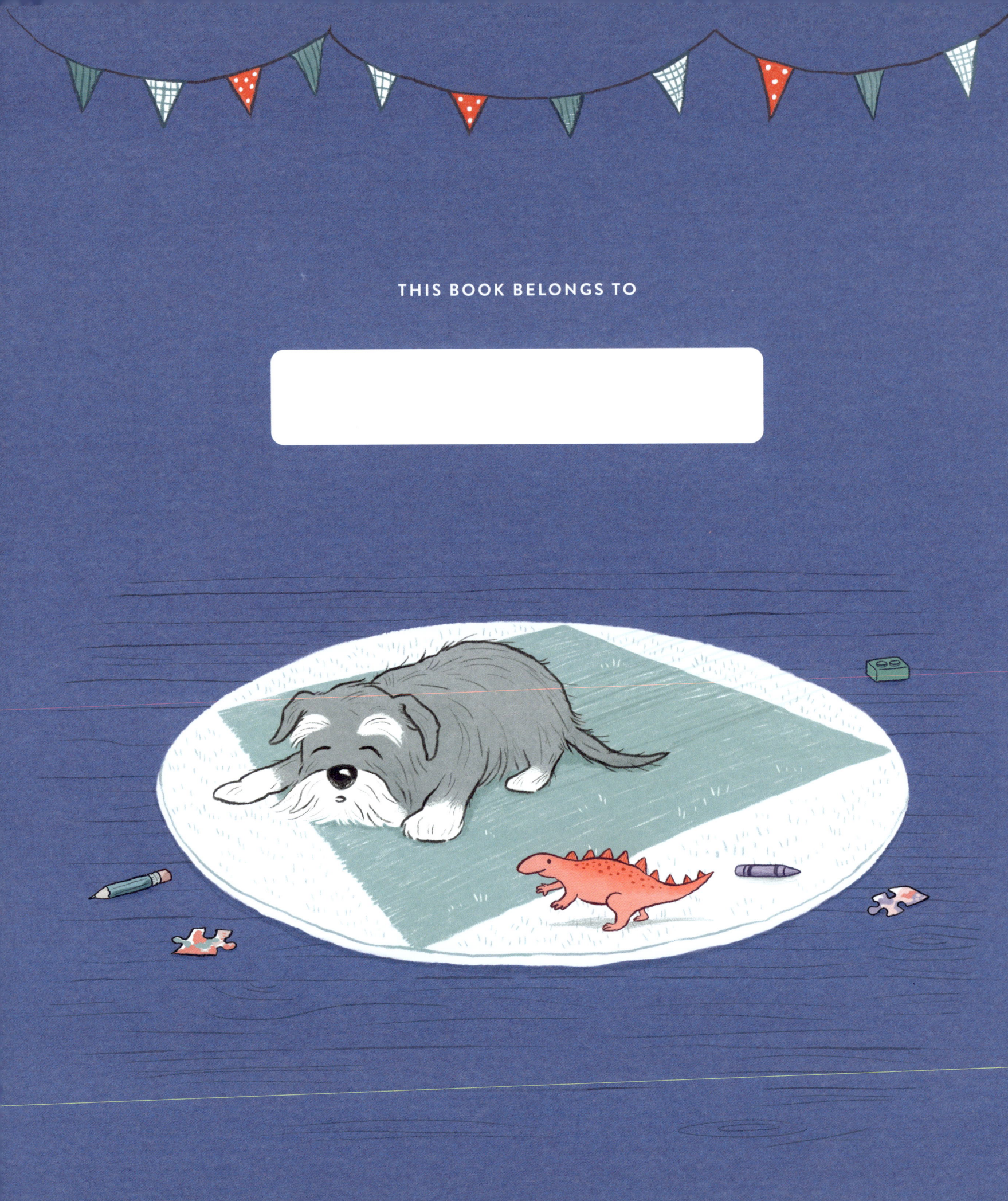

THIS BOOK BELONGS TO

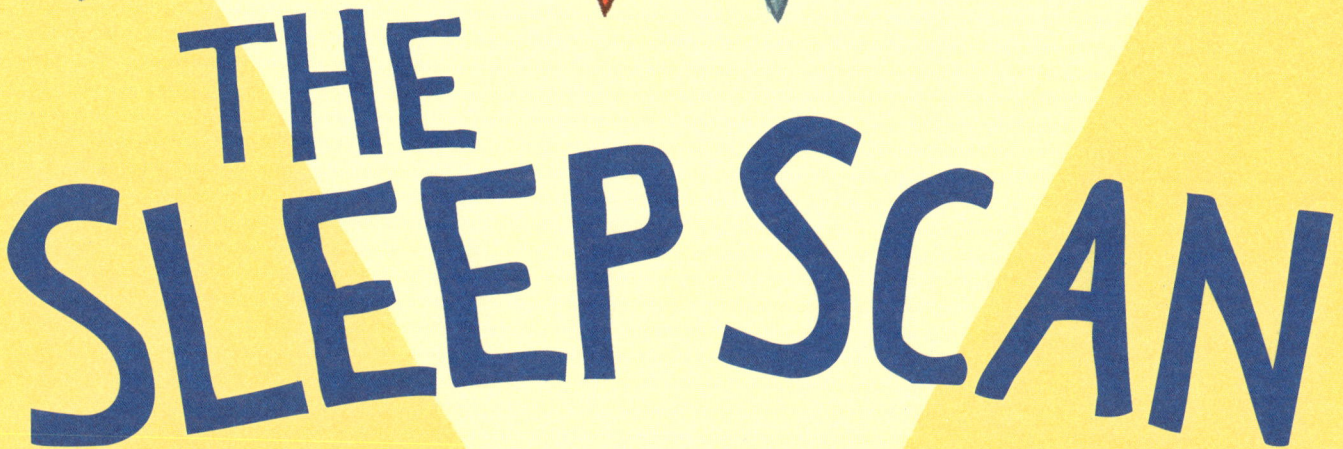

# THE SLEEP SCAN

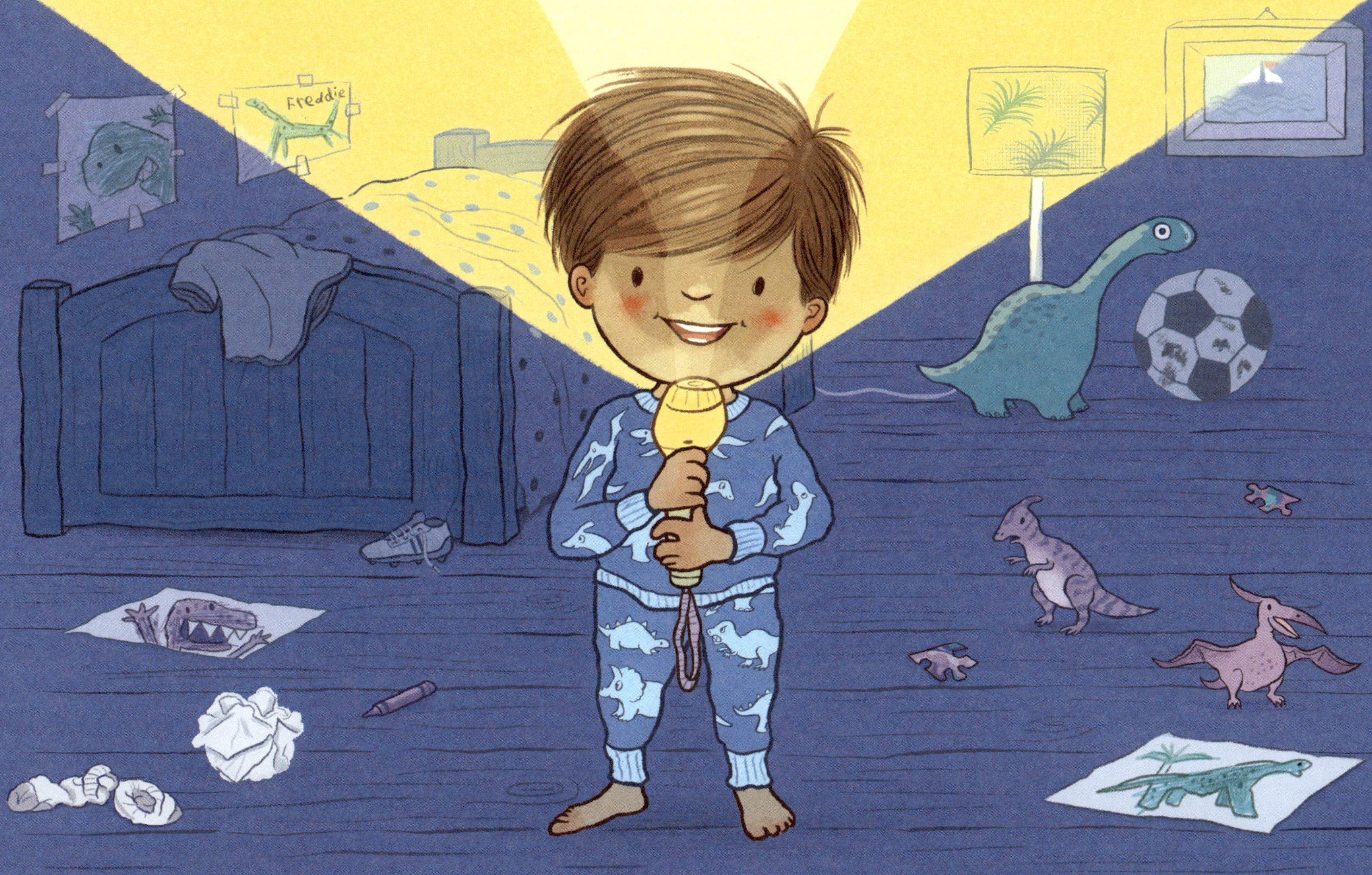

NIALL BRESLIN
ILLUSTRATED BY SHEENA DEMPSEY

GILL BOOKS

Gill Books
Hume Avenue
Park West
Dublin 12
www.gillbooks.ie

Gill Books is an imprint of M.H. Gill and Co.

Text © Niall Breslin 2022, 2023
Illustrations © Sheena Dempsey 2022, 2023
First published in 2022. This paperback edition published 2023.

978 07171 9744 6

Designed by www.grahamthew.com
Printed and bound by L&C Printing Group, Poland
This book is typeset in Archer.

*The paper used in this book comes from the wood pulp of sustainably managed forests.*

All rights reserved.
No part of this publication may be copied, reproduced or transmitted in any form or by any means, without written permission of the publishers.

A CIP catalogue record for this book is available from the British Library.

5 4 3 2 1

## A NOTE FOR PARENTS

Well, that was a bumpy few years!

I've spent much of the last few months trying to get my head around what we all went through. I often think, *How must our young folk be processing it all?*

And it can be hard for us adults at times when we try to help the kids in our lives make sense of something that we can't really get our heads around either.

Personally speaking, I feel quite rinsed, exhausted and courting a constant sense of hyper-vigilance and anxiety. In the past I might have kept ploughing on, in a maze of constant distraction, pretending that I was okay. But mindfulness has taught me to sit with this discomfort. Observe it. Don't push it away or repress it. And in doing that, I started to realise that the way I am feeling is a perfectly healthy human response to a crisis. That it's exactly how I should be feeling. And it's important that the kids in our lives have space to do this too: to communicate and express these emotions.

Another thing I noticed during the pandemic was that this hyper-vigilant default setting I was in was playing havoc with my sleep patterns. I would go to bed full of thoughts and energy and then just stare at the ceiling – or worse, at my phone. My mind felt as though it was so dynamic that sleep was the last thing it wanted to do. I had to make changes.

And so I worked on my evening routine. I avoided the news, social media and bright lights. I tend to meditate in the mornings before my day starts, but I started to practise the body scan in the evenings, to tune my body down and get it out of that hyper-vigilant state of worry and rumination, and into a state of presence, awareness and rest.

In time, changes like this became habits and my sleep patterns returned to a normal, healthy state.

When I sleep well, or even rest well, my mental and physical bandwidth widens. I have the capacity to cope with so much more.

We all know the importance of sleep, but it's crucial for kids, especially as their brains develop. Good sleep helps their mood, behaviour, growth, resilience and memory. Kids nowadays have so much going on. Their minds can sometimes get too busy. Teaching them how to become present and aware through mindfulness helps them to slow down a racing mind, so that they can rest and sleep and build up all the energy that they need to play, learn and have fun each day. Teaching them the habit of tuning down each night with a technique like the body scan is a gift they will always be thankful for.

Here are a few other tried and tested sleep tips to help bedtime go more smoothly. Good luck!

Bressie x

•

- Start to get your child ready for bed at the same time every night.

- Encourage some physical activity in the afternoon or early evening, before starting to slow things down before bedtime.

- Make sure your child has eaten some supper and that they are not hungry.

- Switch off all screens at least an hour before bed, and keep these out of the bedroom.

- A warm bath before bed can help relax children, as can a quiet family activity, such as reading a short story together, or singing a lullaby.

- To help them settle, dim the bedroom lights and switch on a night light if your child is afraid of the dark.

- Some children like to have a stuffed toy or security blanket.

- A mindfulness technique like the body scan can really help as well.

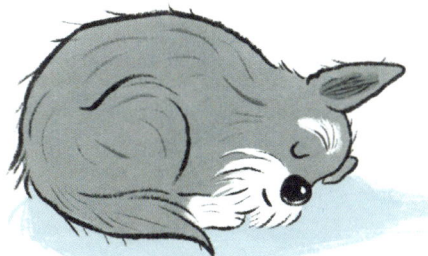

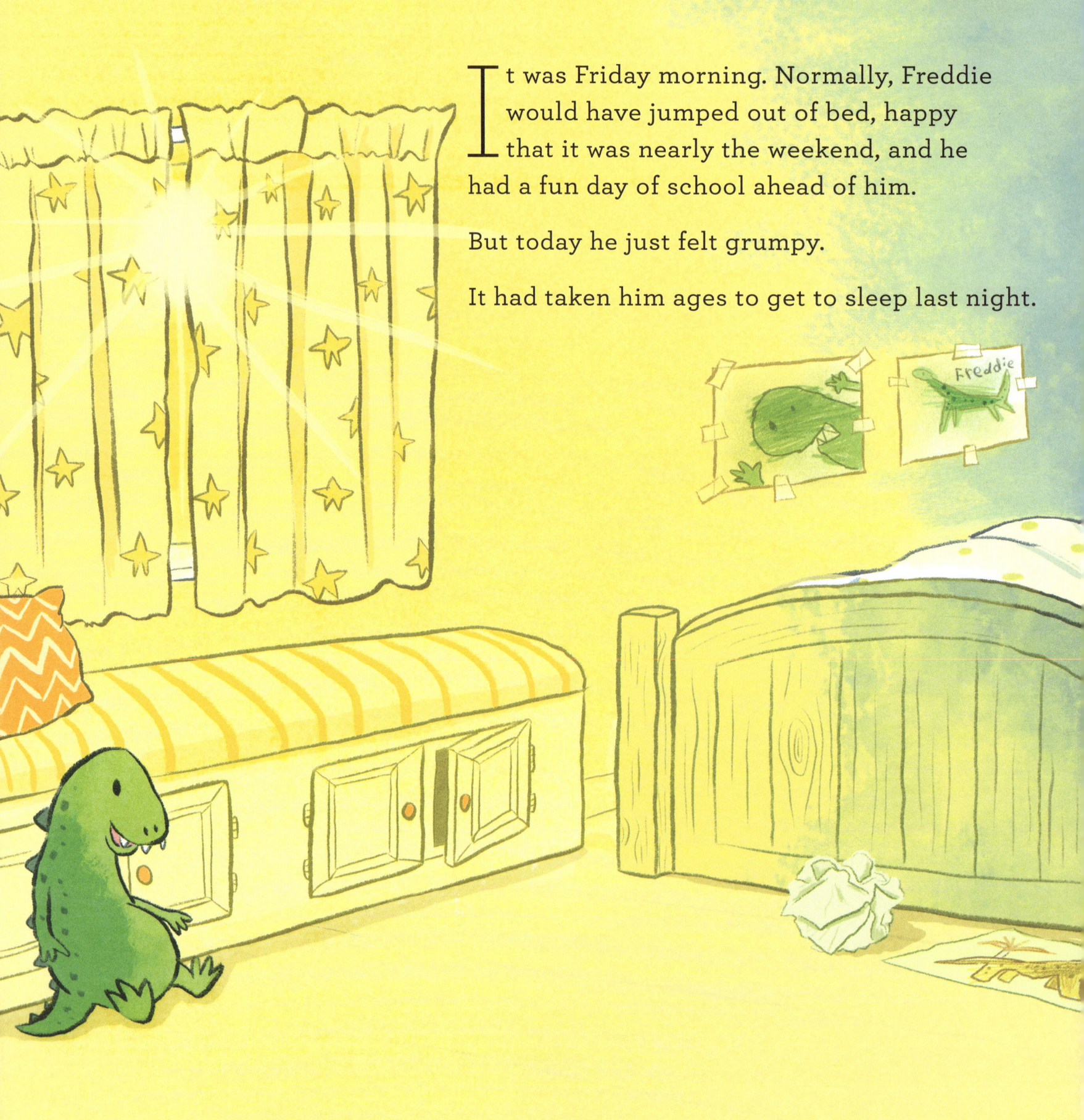

It was Friday morning. Normally, Freddie would have jumped out of bed, happy that it was nearly the weekend, and he had a fun day of school ahead of him.

But today he just felt grumpy.

It had taken him ages to get to sleep last night.

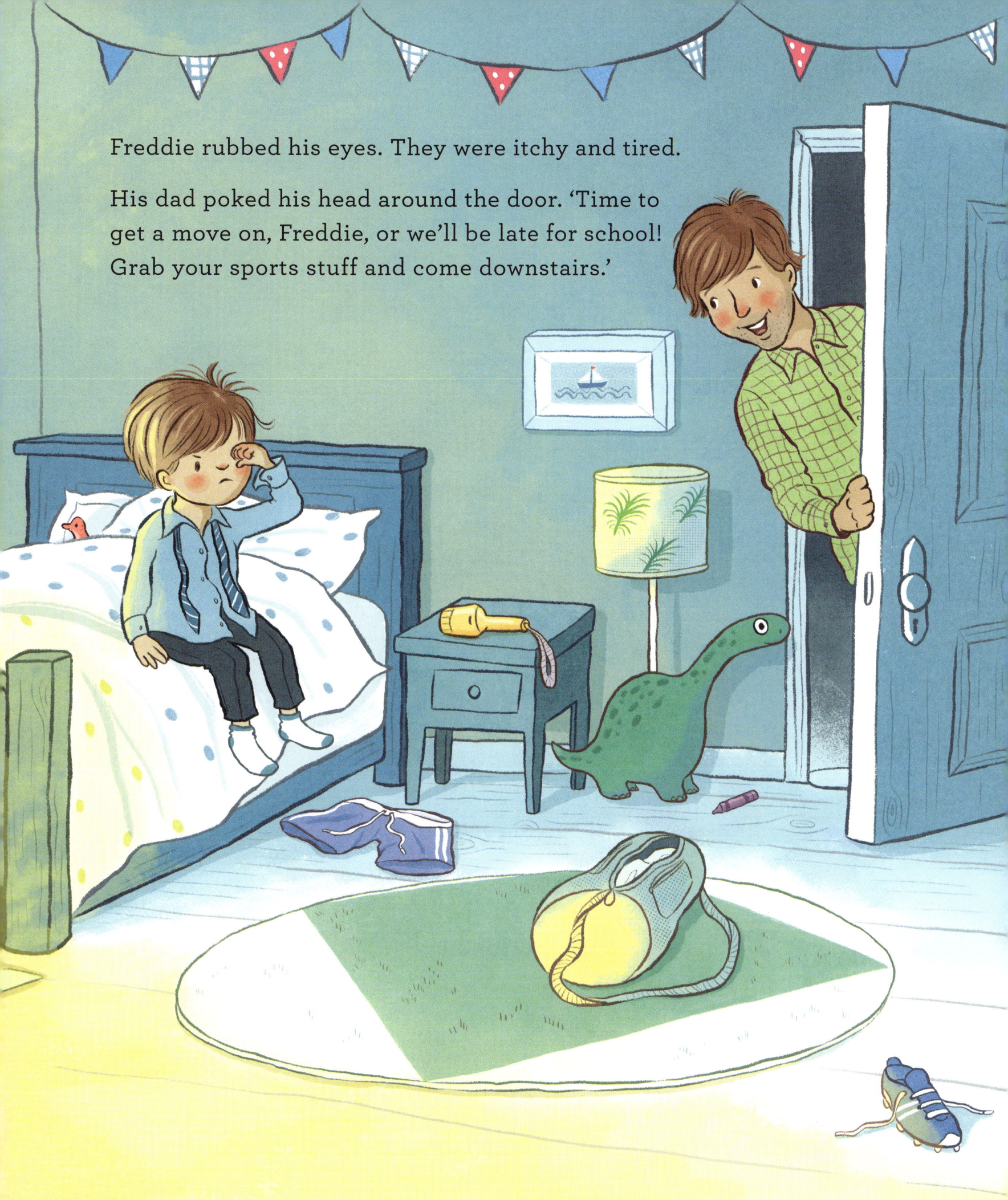

Freddie rubbed his eyes. They were itchy and tired.

His dad poked his head around the door. 'Time to get a move on, Freddie, or we'll be late for school! Grab your sports stuff and come downstairs.'

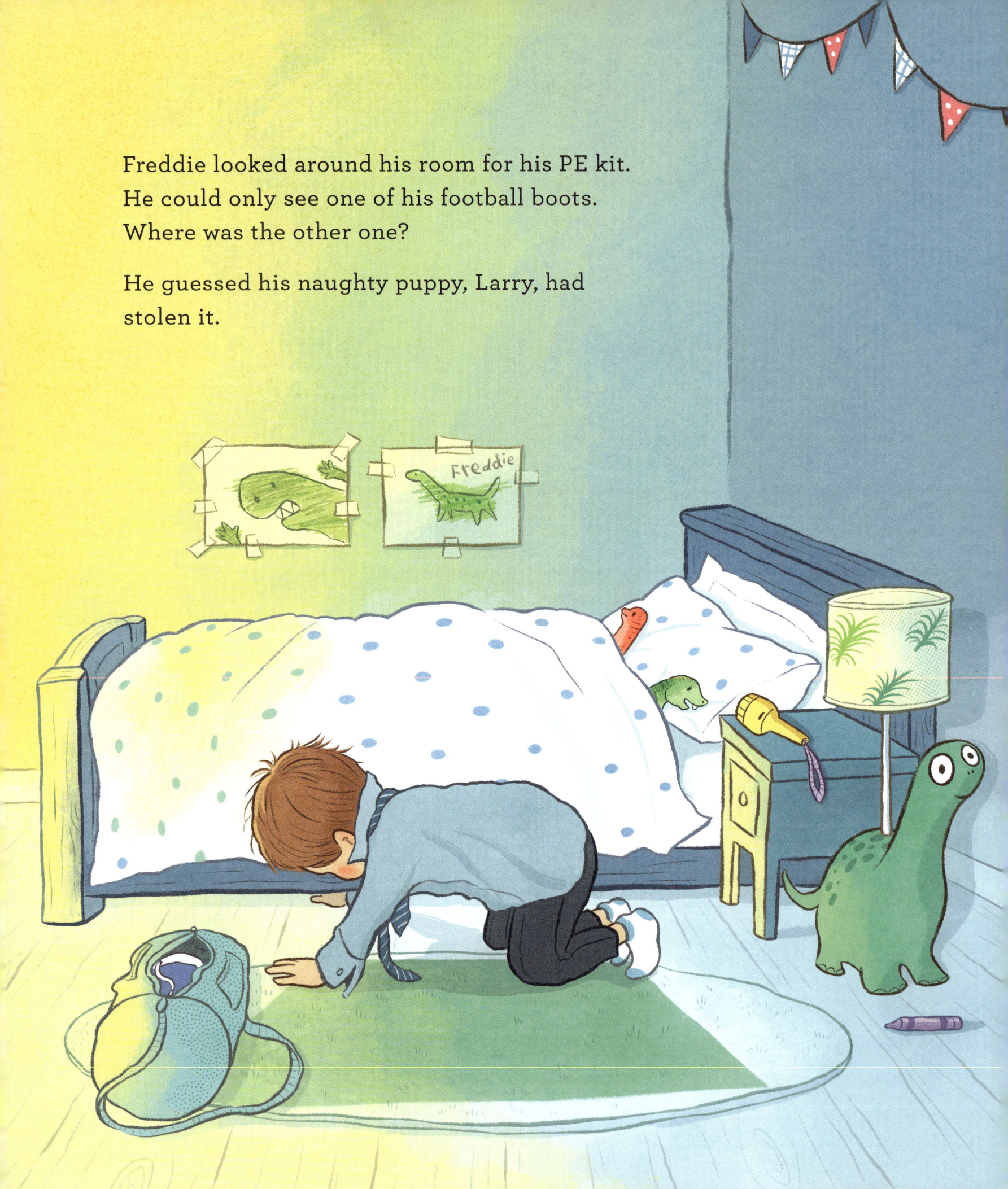

Freddie looked around his room for his PE kit. He could only see one of his football boots. Where was the other one?

He guessed his naughty puppy, Larry, had stolen it.

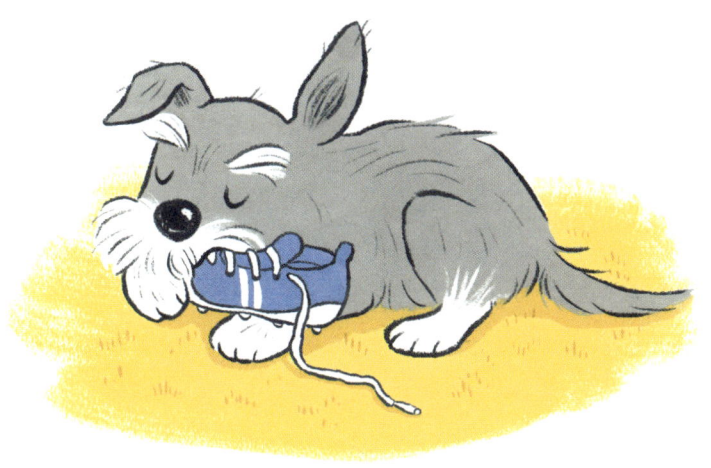

Freddie was right. Larry was chewing his boot out on the landing.

Freddie tried to grab it, but Larry ran off, thinking it was a game.

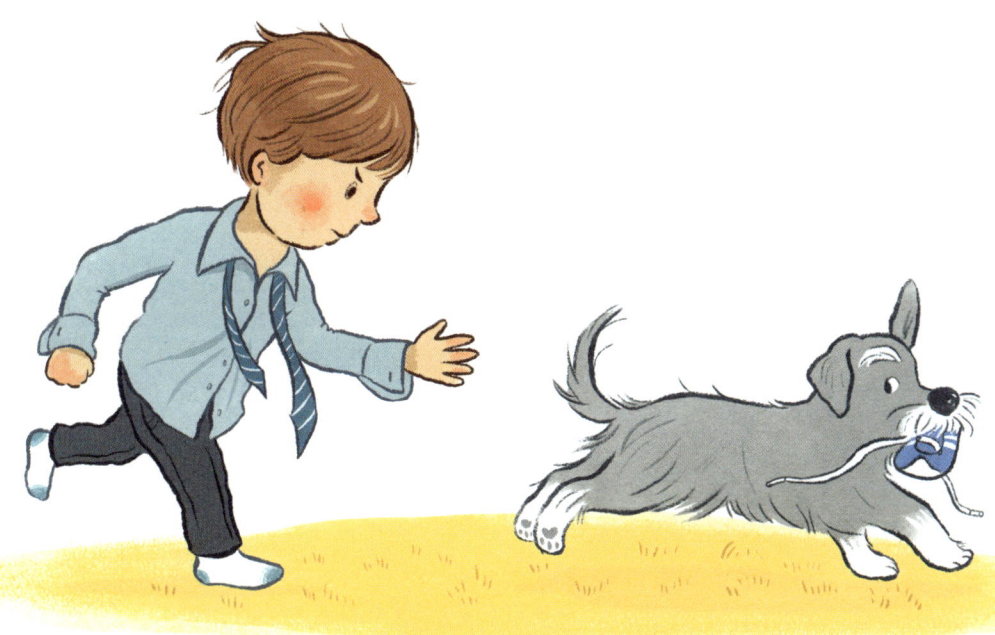

At last Freddie managed to get the boot back, and stomped downstairs, leaving Larry wondering why his friend didn't want to play this morning.

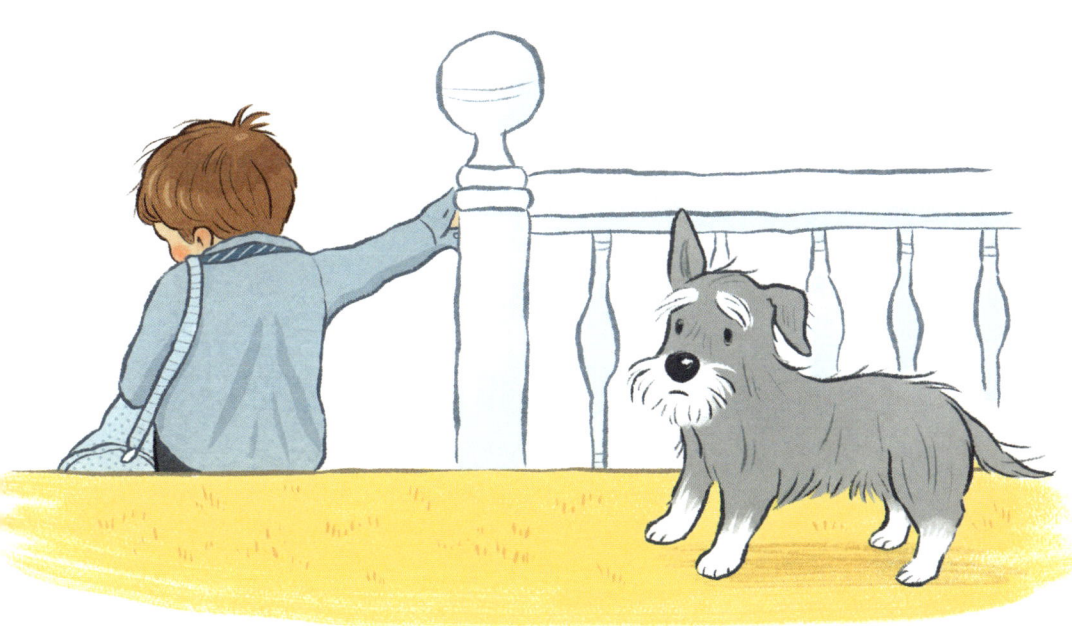

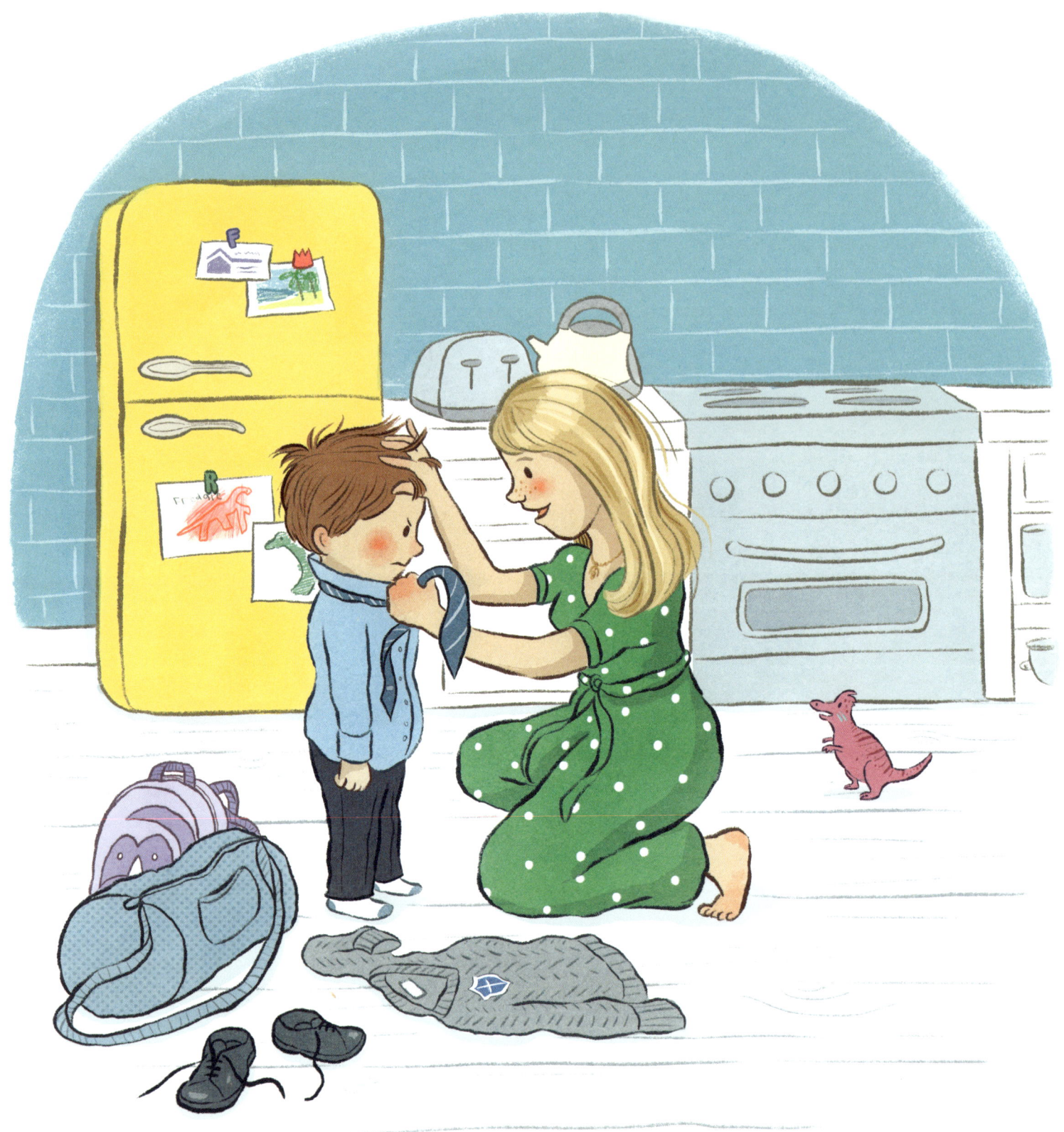

'Ah, there you are at last, Freddie,' said Mum, as he came into the kitchen.

She helped Freddie with his shirt and tie and then ruffled his hair. This normally made him smile, but not today.

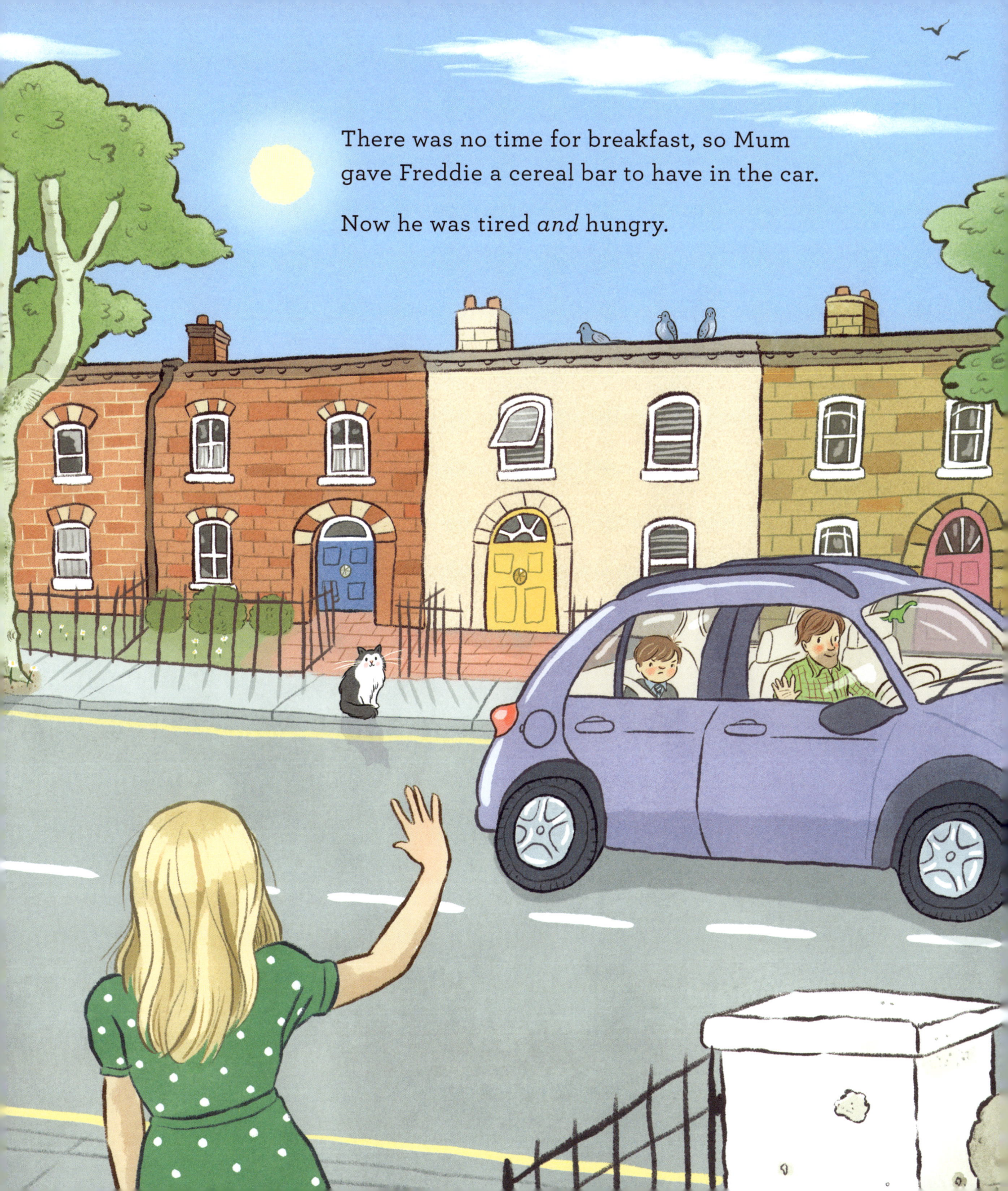

Things at school didn't get much better.

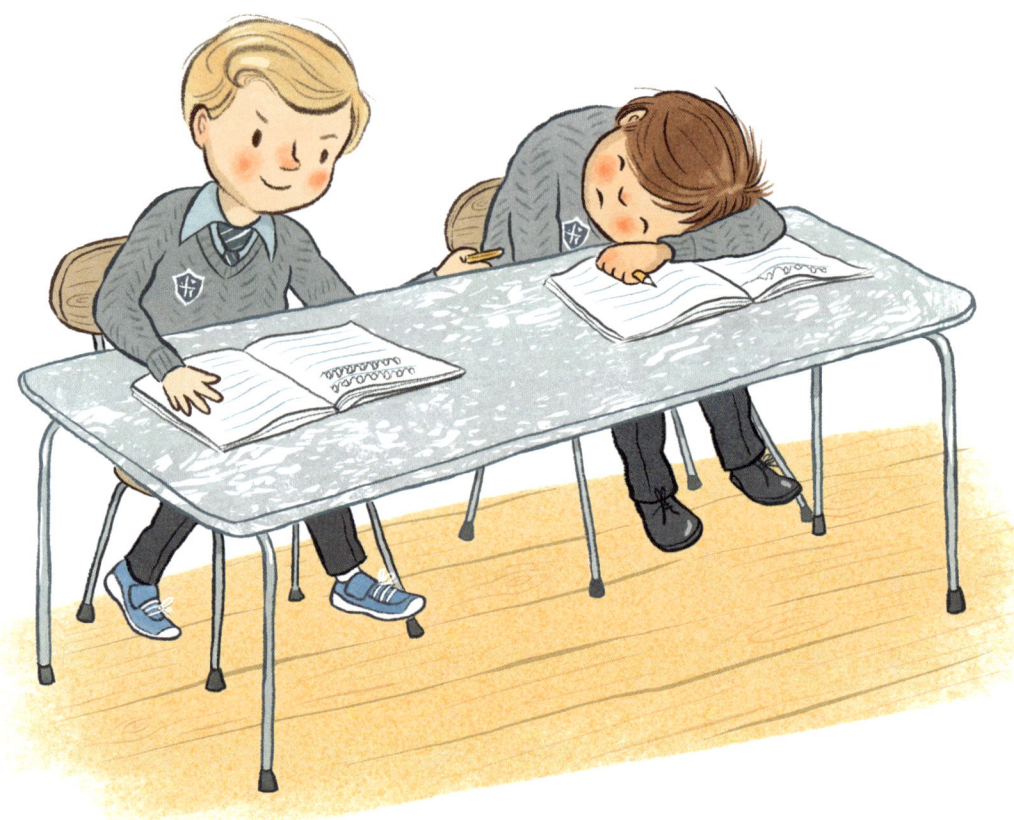

Freddie nodded off in class, and when his best friend, Ben, poked him with a pencil to wake him up, Freddie jumped out of his chair in surprise.

Their teacher told them both off for messing about.

Then Freddie spilled paint all over himself during art.

Being tired was making him clumsy.

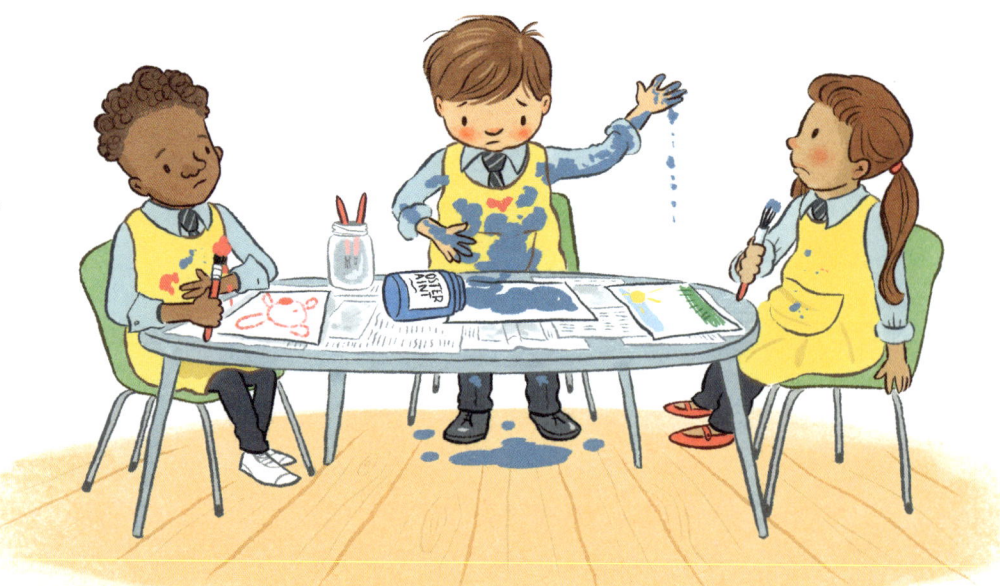

It took so long to clean the paint off that Freddie was late for lunch. The canteen had run out of his favourite strawberry yoghurt and he had to have a piece of fruit instead.

'Today is a bad day!' he thought.

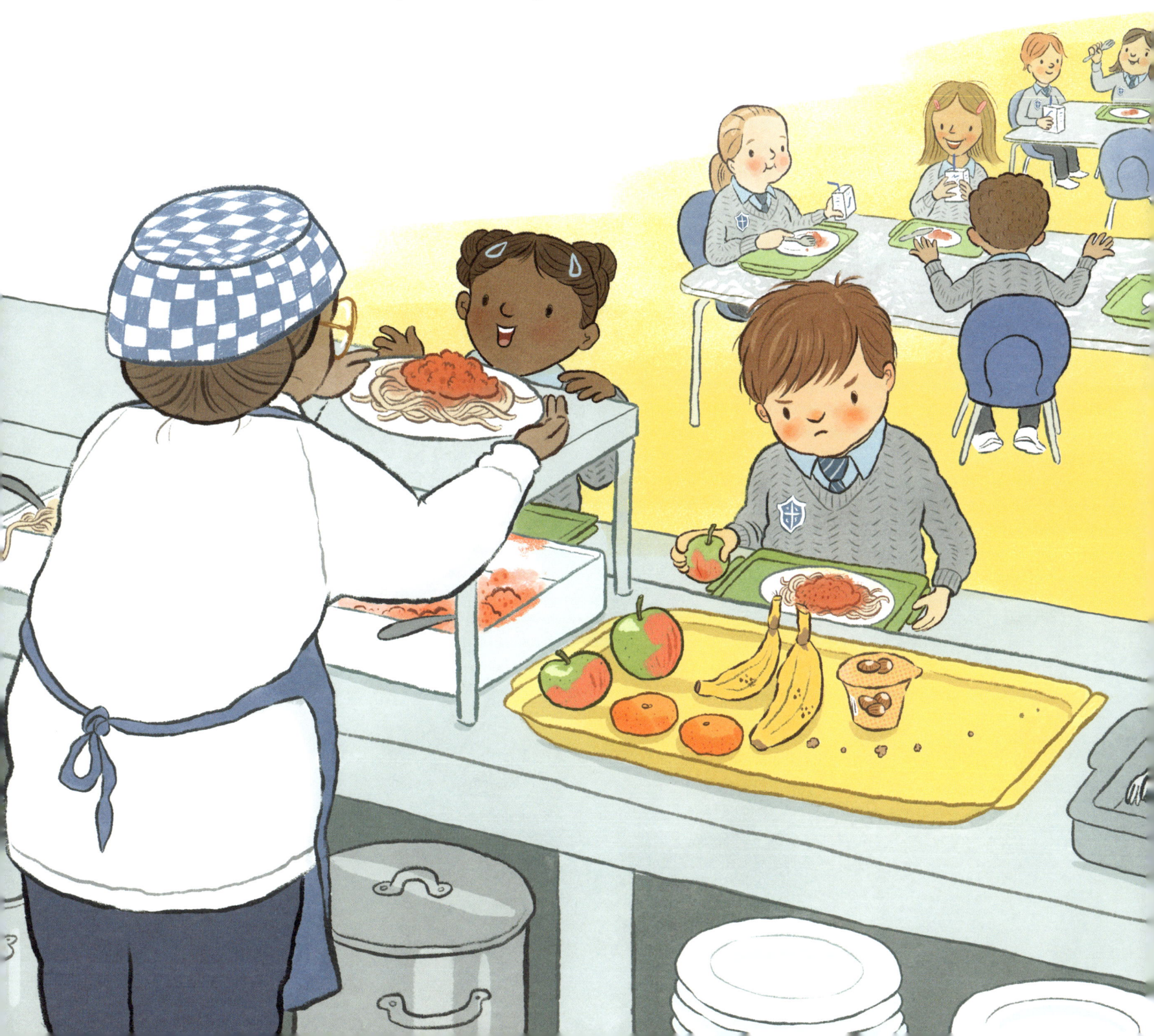

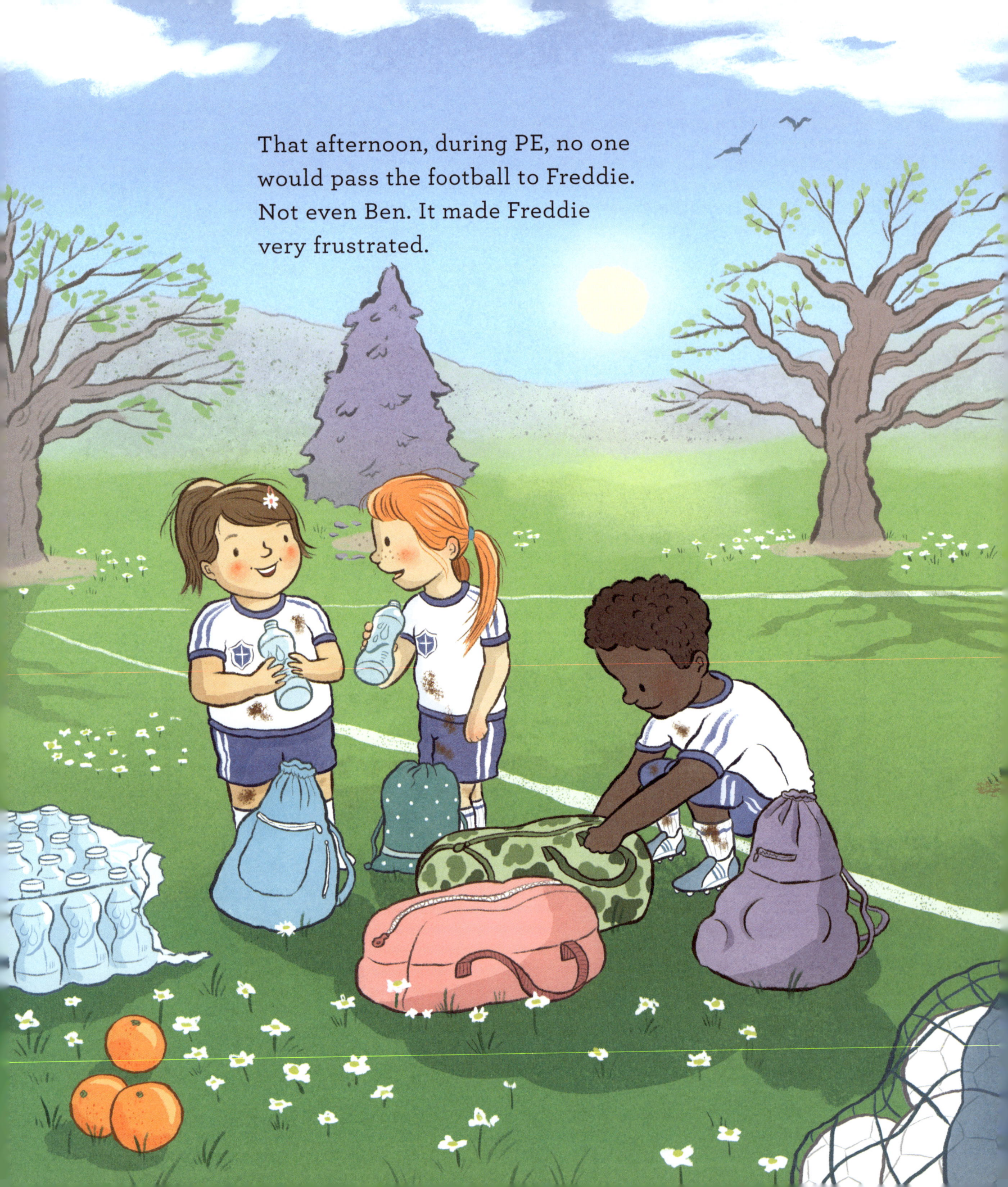

That afternoon, during PE, no one would pass the football to Freddie. Not even Ben. It made Freddie very frustrated.

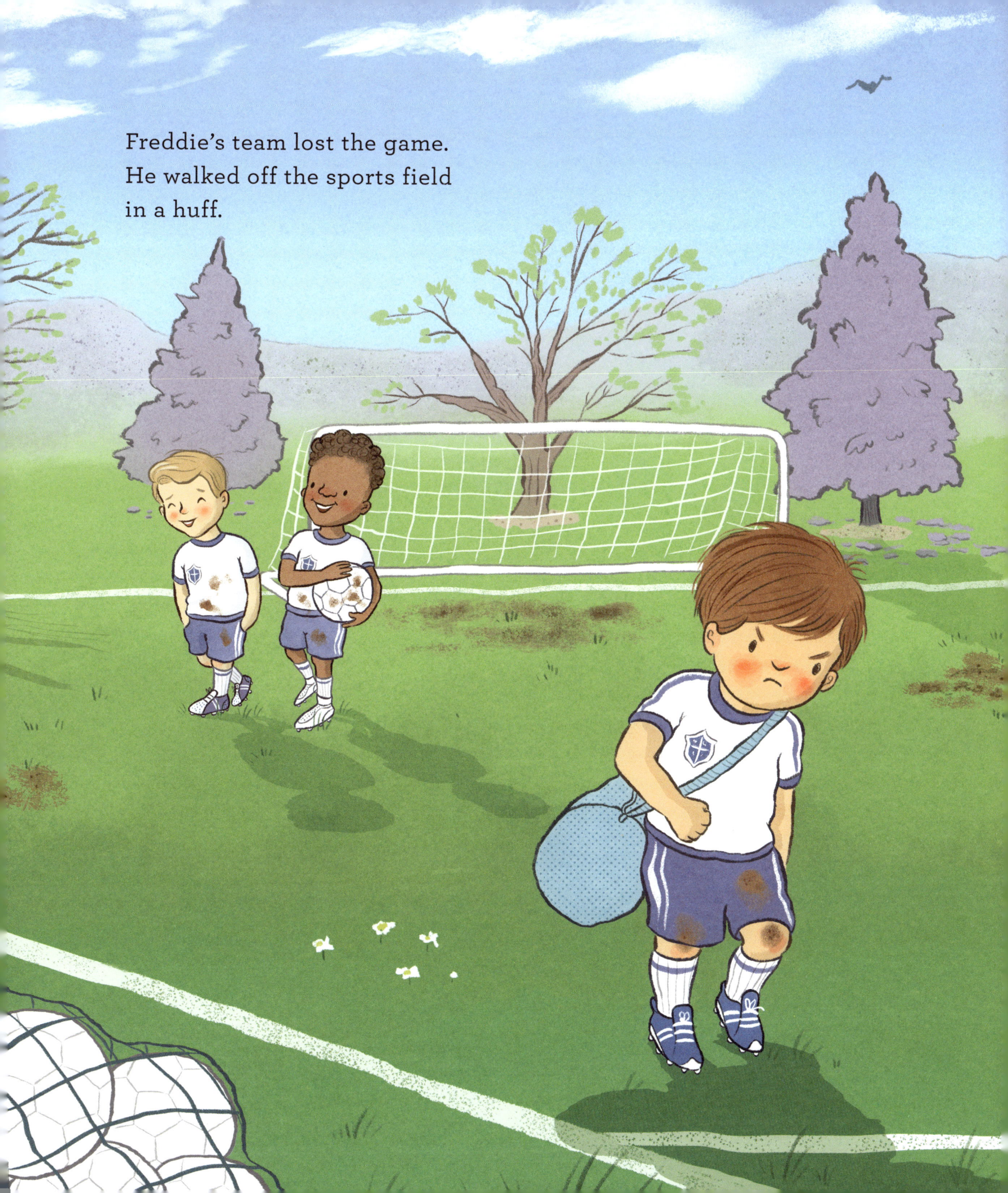

Freddie's team lost the game. He walked off the sports field in a huff.

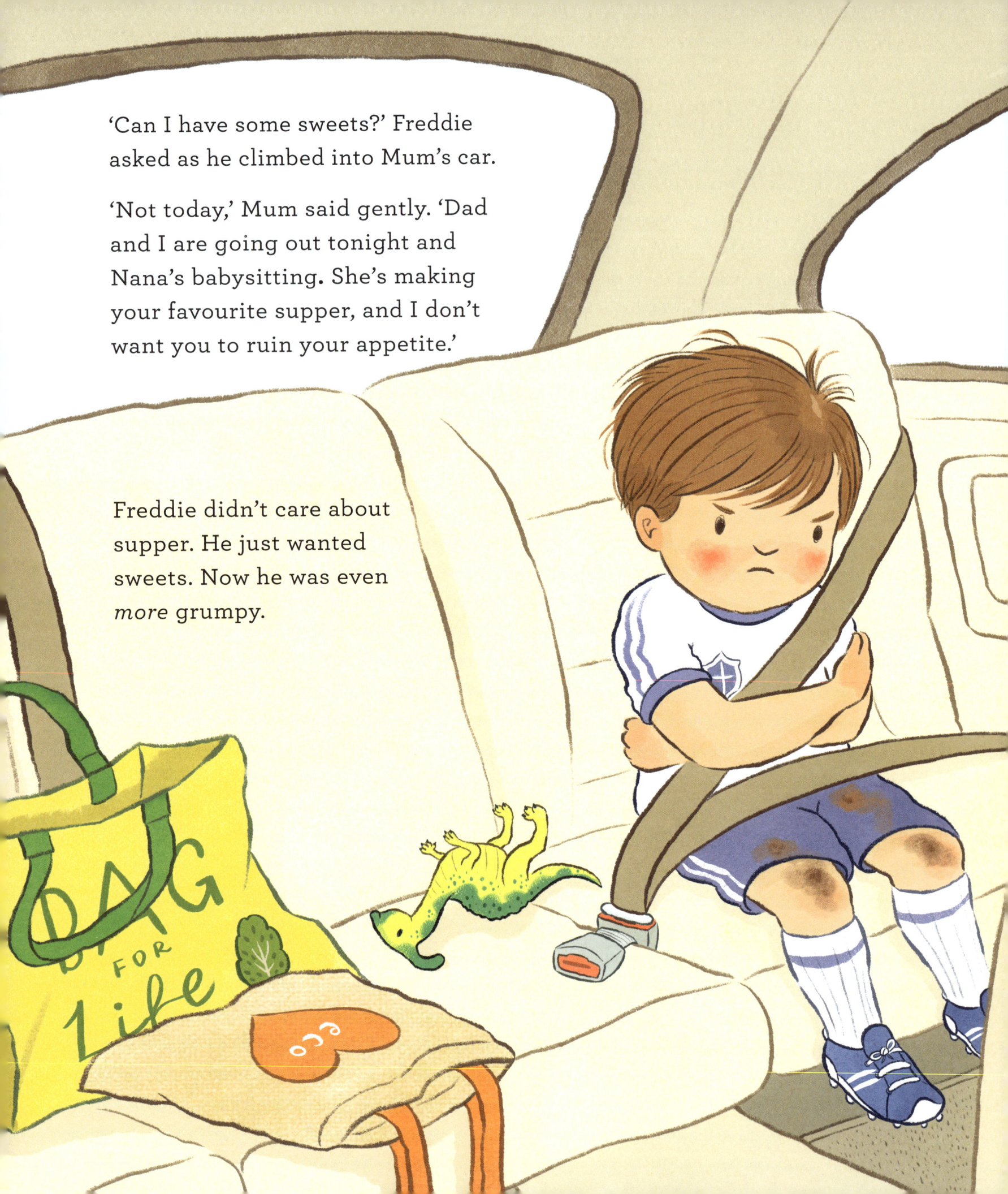

'Can I have some sweets?' Freddie asked as he climbed into Mum's car.

'Not today,' Mum said gently. 'Dad and I are going out tonight and Nana's babysitting. She's making your favourite supper, and I don't want you to ruin your appetite.'

Freddie didn't care about supper. He just wanted sweets. Now he was even *more* grumpy.

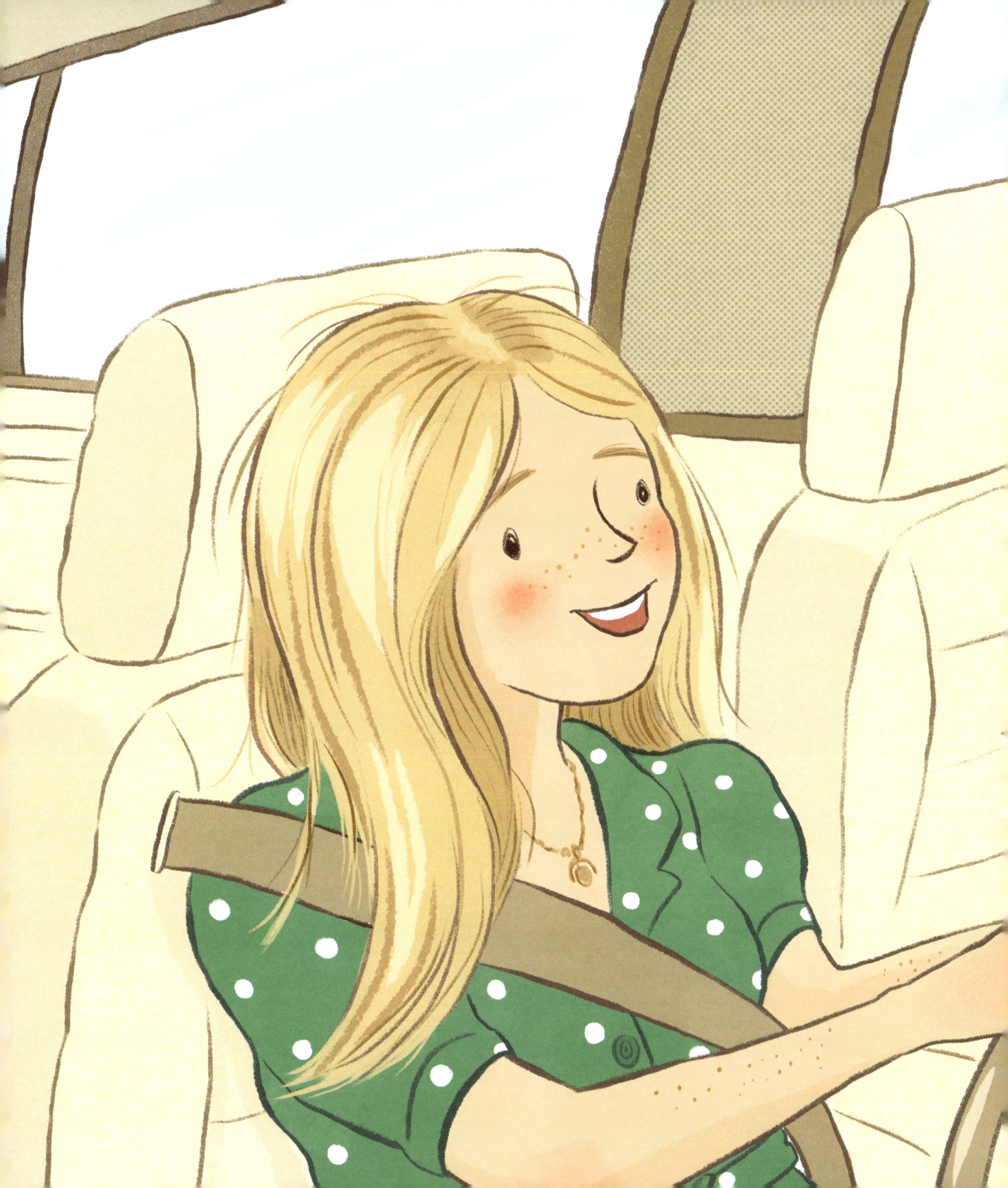

When Freddie got home, even one of Nana's world-famous Nana hugs didn't help.

After supper, Nana suggested they play a board game before bed. But Freddie didn't want to.

He didn't want to play with his dinosaurs either.

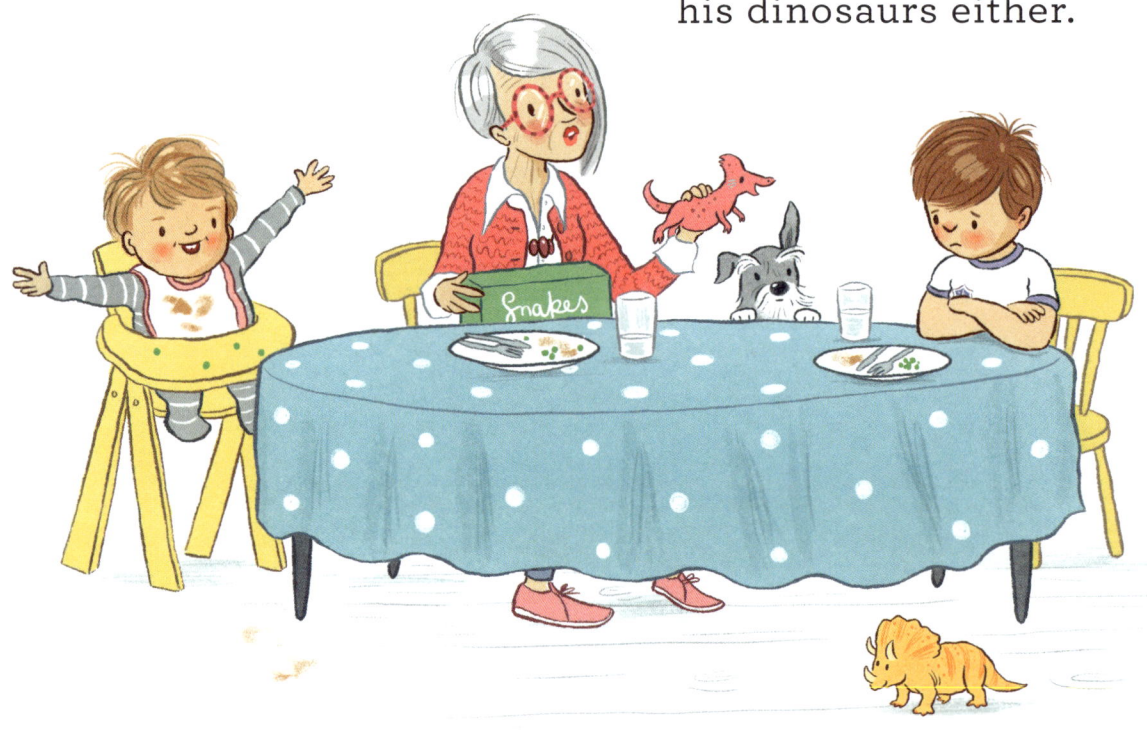

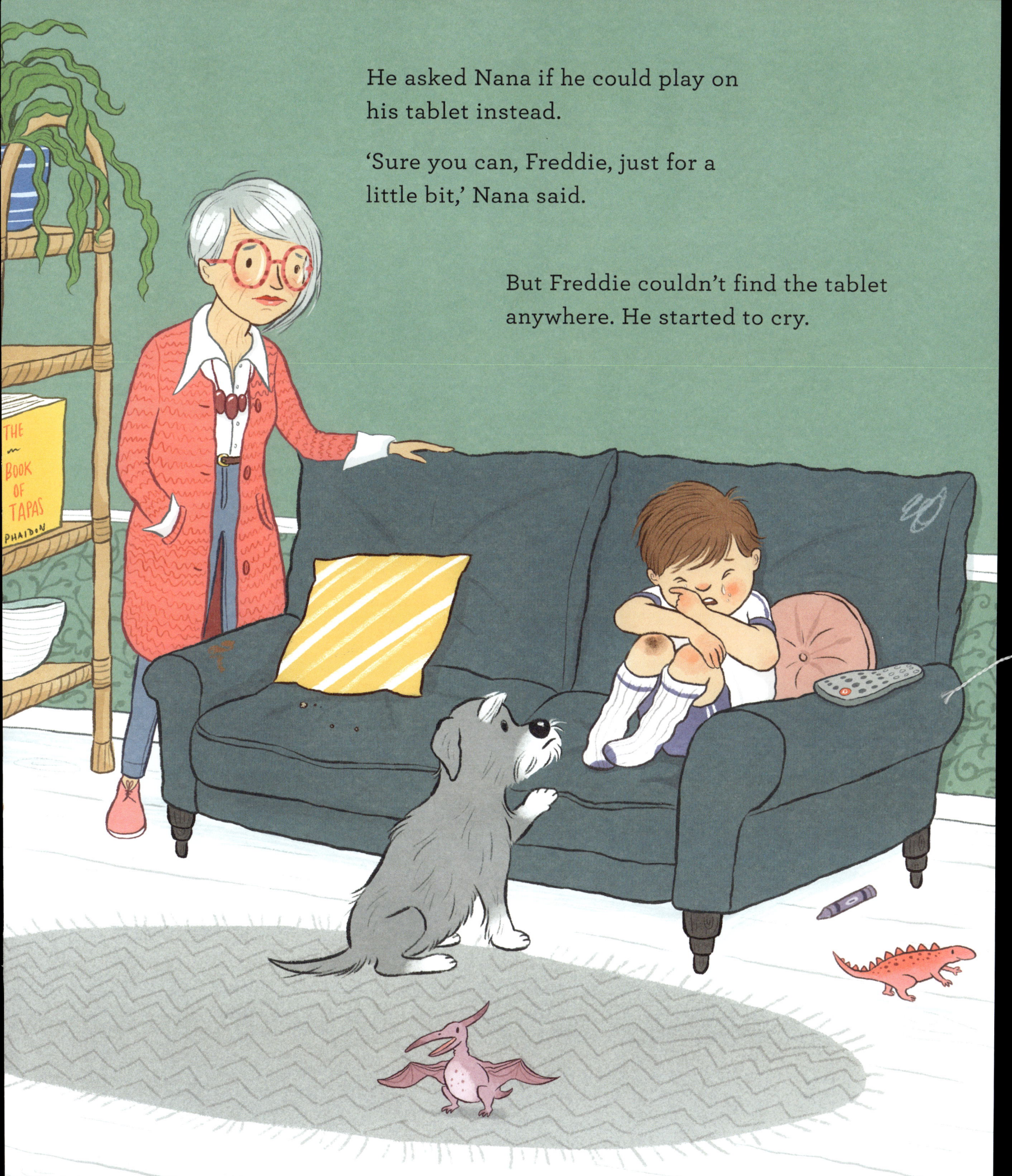

He asked Nana if he could play on his tablet instead.

'Sure you can, Freddie, just for a little bit,' Nana said.

But Freddie couldn't find the tablet anywhere. He started to cry.

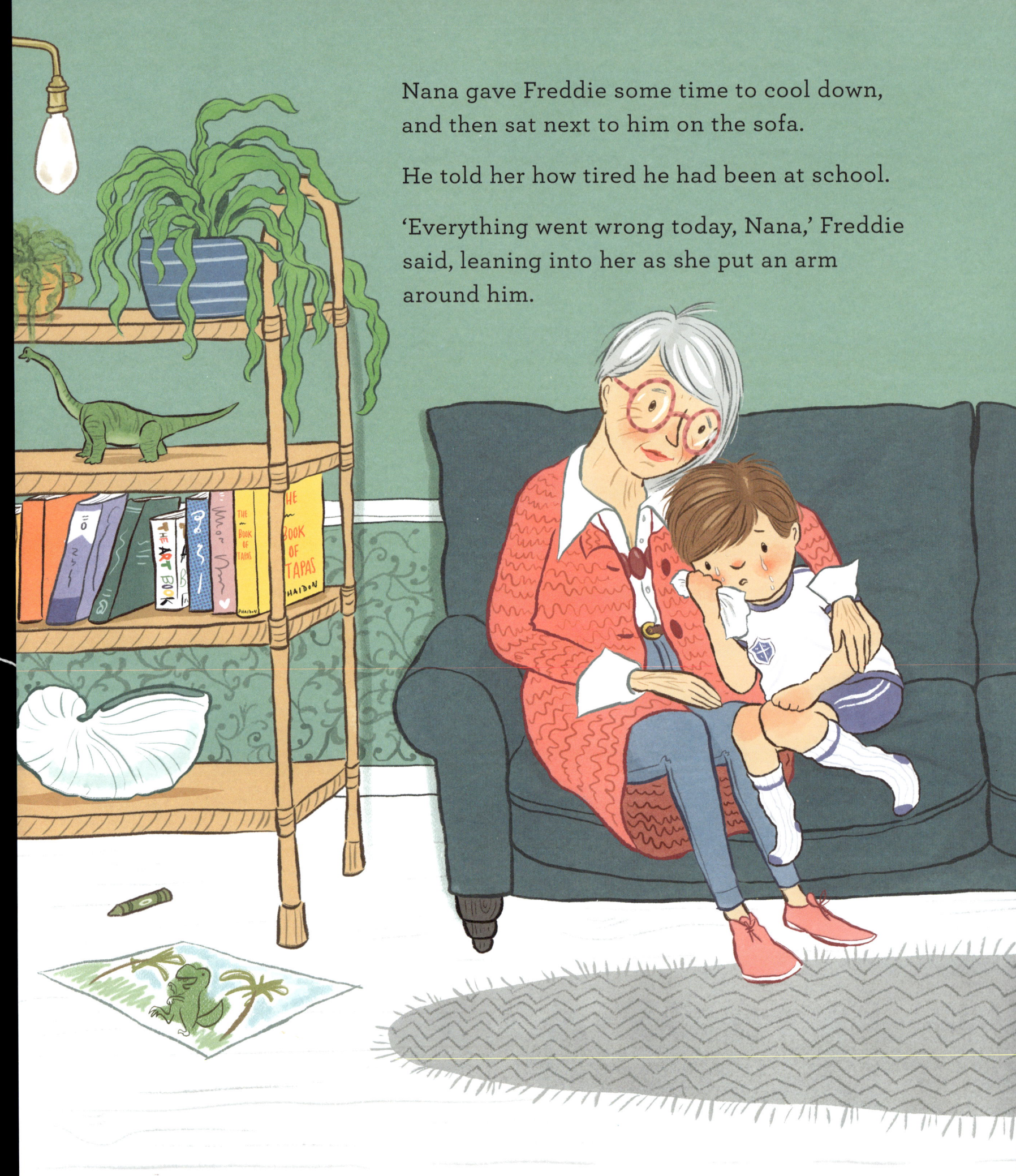

Nana gave Freddie some time to cool down, and then sat next to him on the sofa.

He told her how tired he had been at school.

'Everything went wrong today, Nana,' Freddie said, leaning into her as she put an arm around him.

Nana smiled. 'Things can feel like a struggle when you're tired. Sleeping well is so important. I have a great trick that helps me when I find it hard to sleep.'

'Really, Nana?' Freddie said. 'Can you teach me it?'

'Of course,' she said. 'If you start getting ready for bed, I'll come up and show you.'

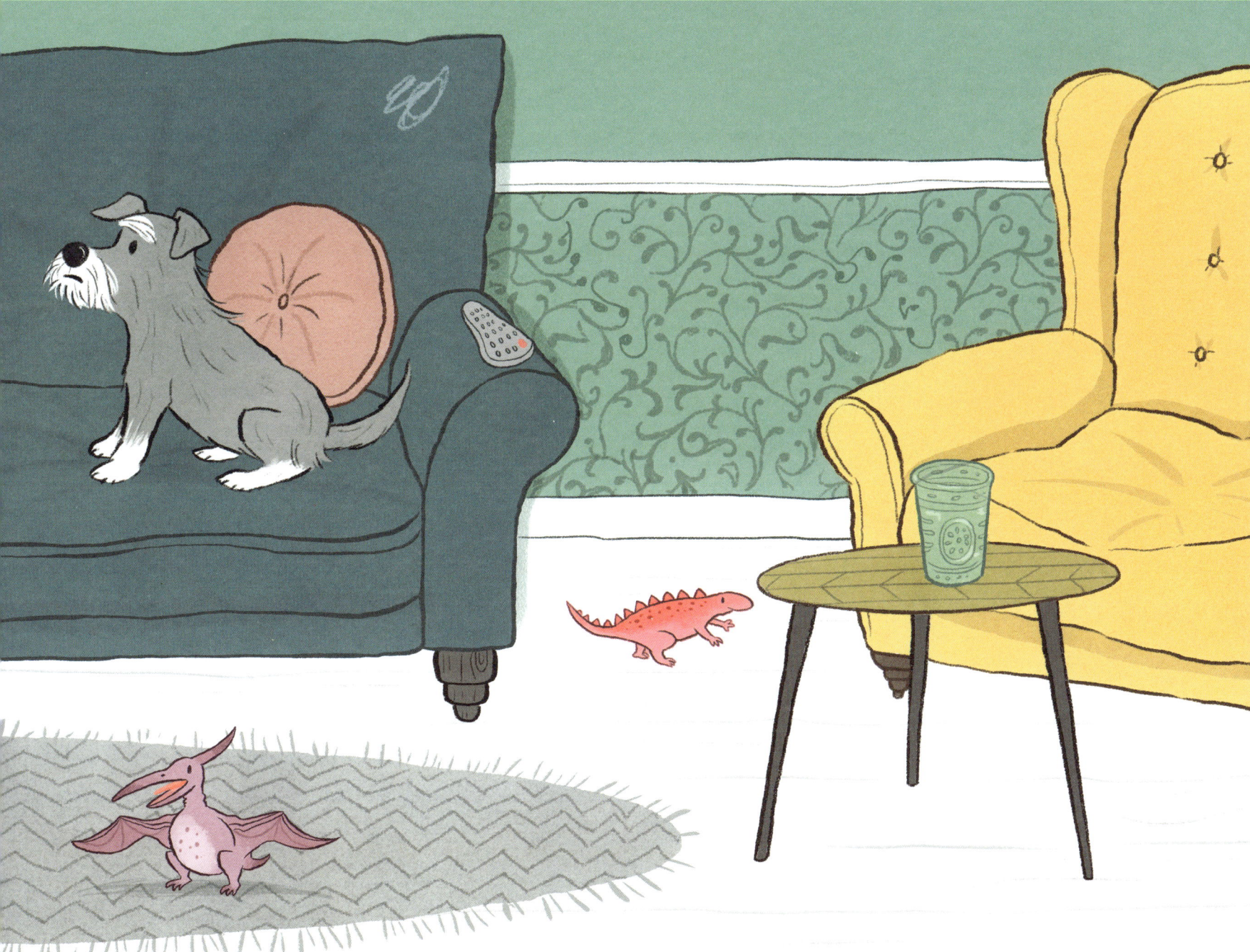

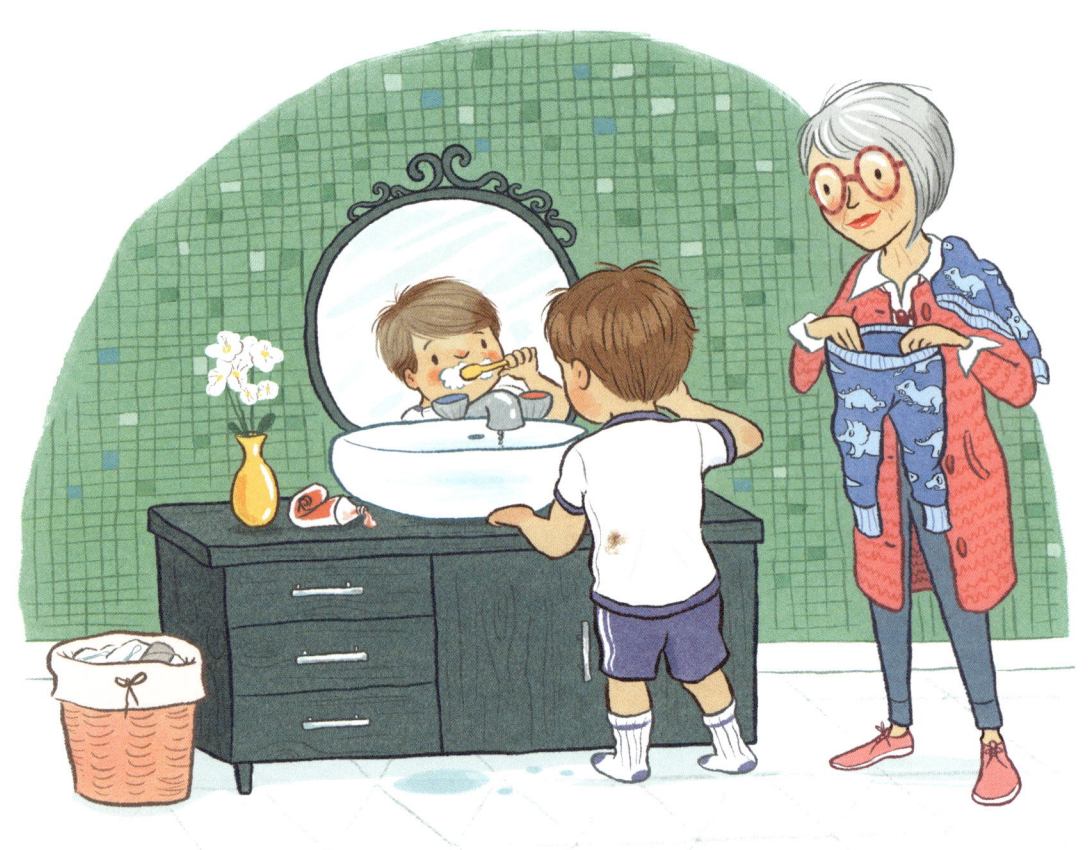

Freddie brushed his teeth and Nana helped him into his pyjamas. She read him a story, and then turned down the lights.

'Remind me what your favourite colour is, Freddie,' she said, sitting on the edge of his bed.

'Umm ... it's green, Nana,' Freddie replied.

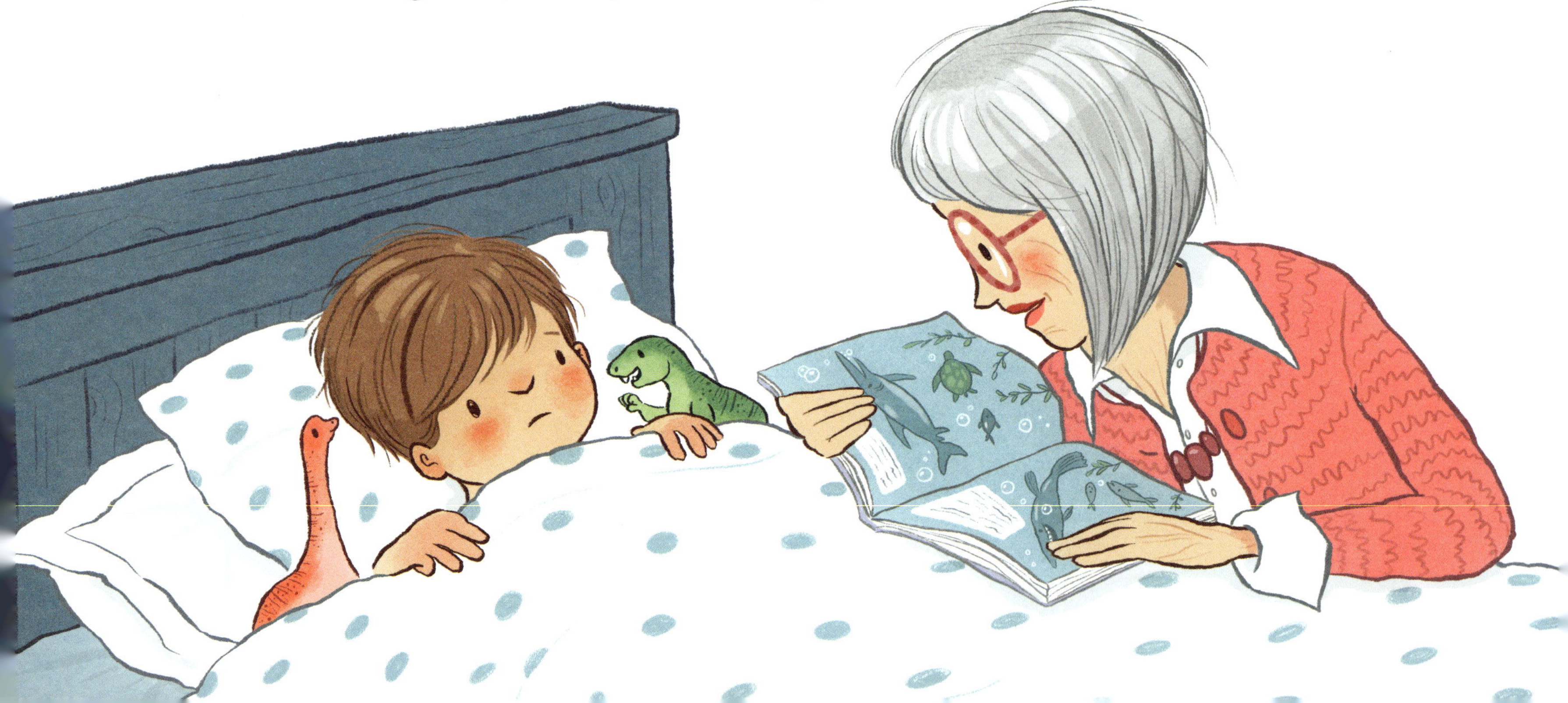

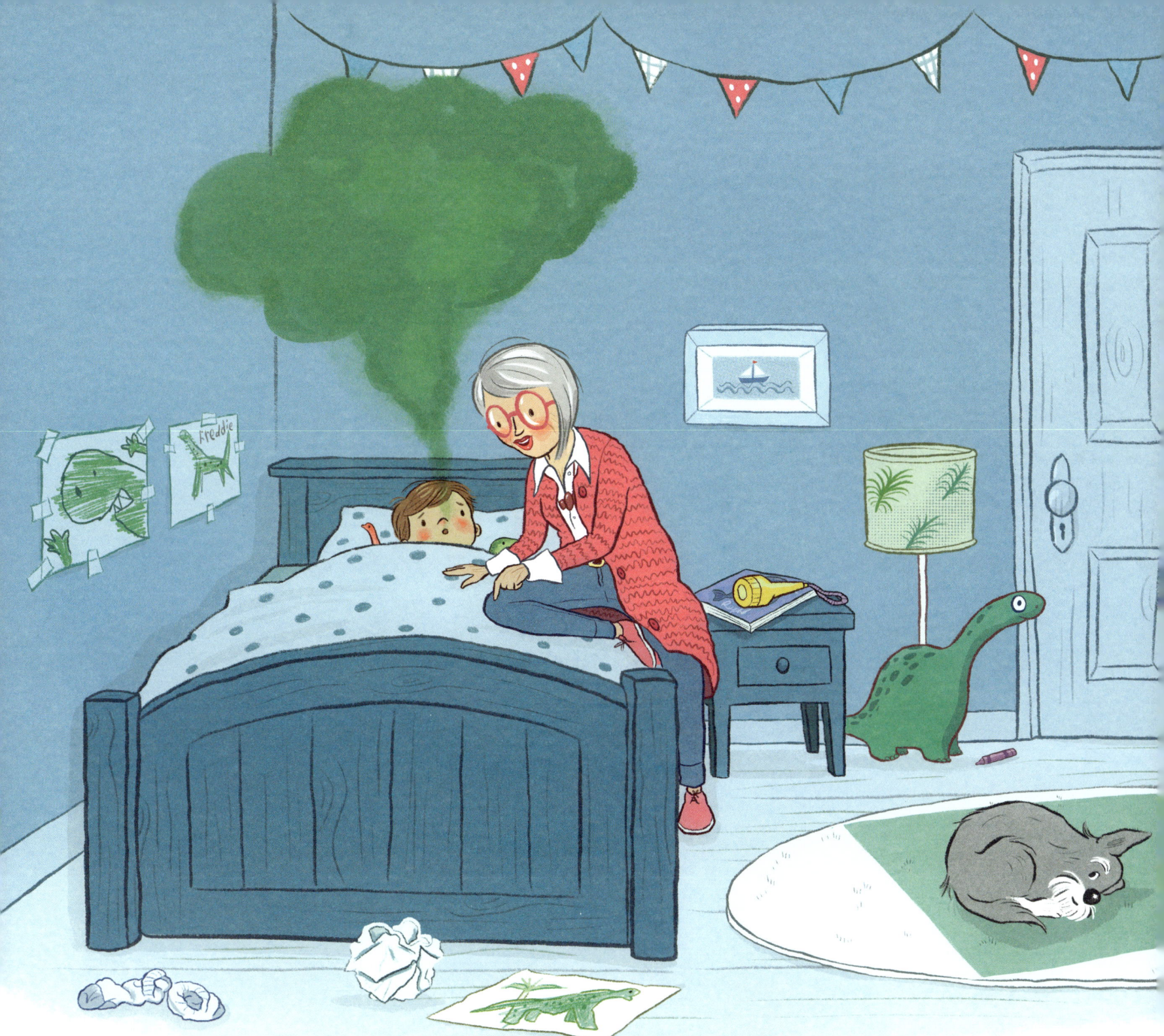

'Right. Place a hand on your belly, and imagine you're breathing the colour green in and out. Slowly in, then slowly out …'

Freddie imagined his room filling up with colour from his breath. He felt like a dragon breathing out smoke!

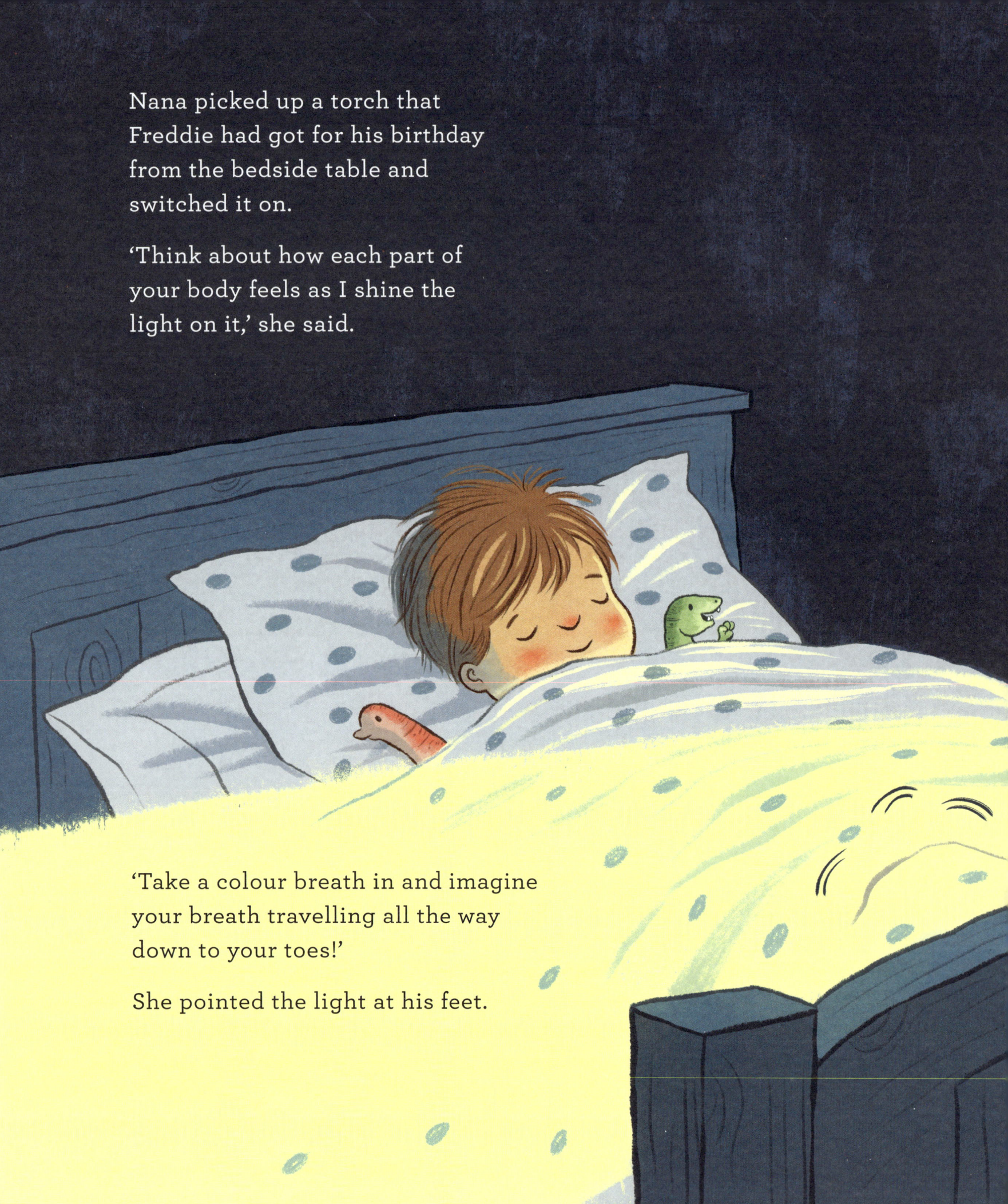

Nana picked up a torch that Freddie had got for his birthday from the bedside table and switched it on.

'Think about how each part of your body feels as I shine the light on it,' she said.

'Take a colour breath in and imagine your breath travelling all the way down to your toes!'

She pointed the light at his feet.

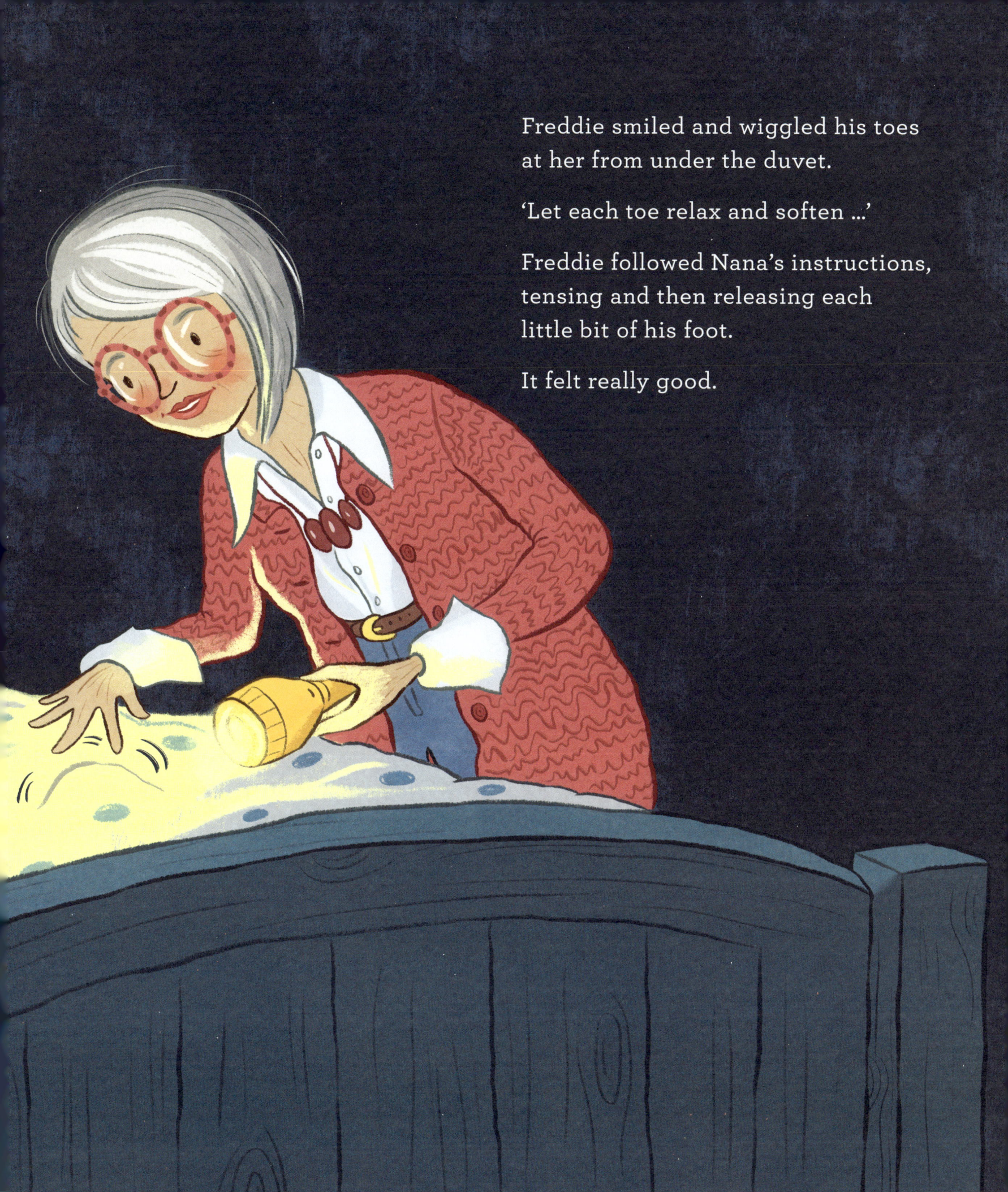

Freddie smiled and wiggled his toes at her from under the duvet.

'Let each toe relax and soften ...'

Freddie followed Nana's instructions, tensing and then releasing each little bit of his foot.

It felt really good.

'Now we're going to move up to your ankles …'

Freddie gently circled his ankles under the covers.

'Then your knees … then your tummy … then your chest …'

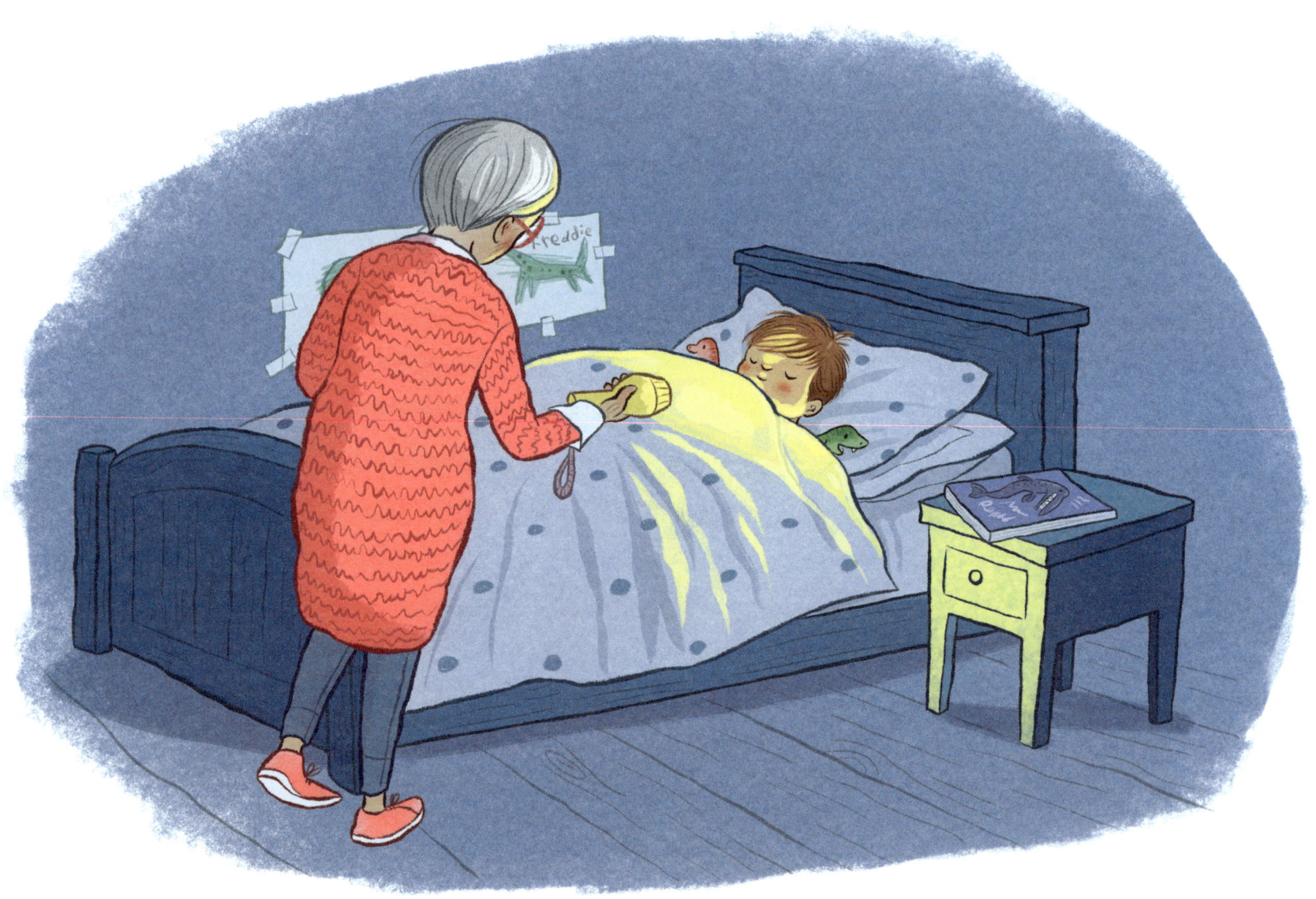

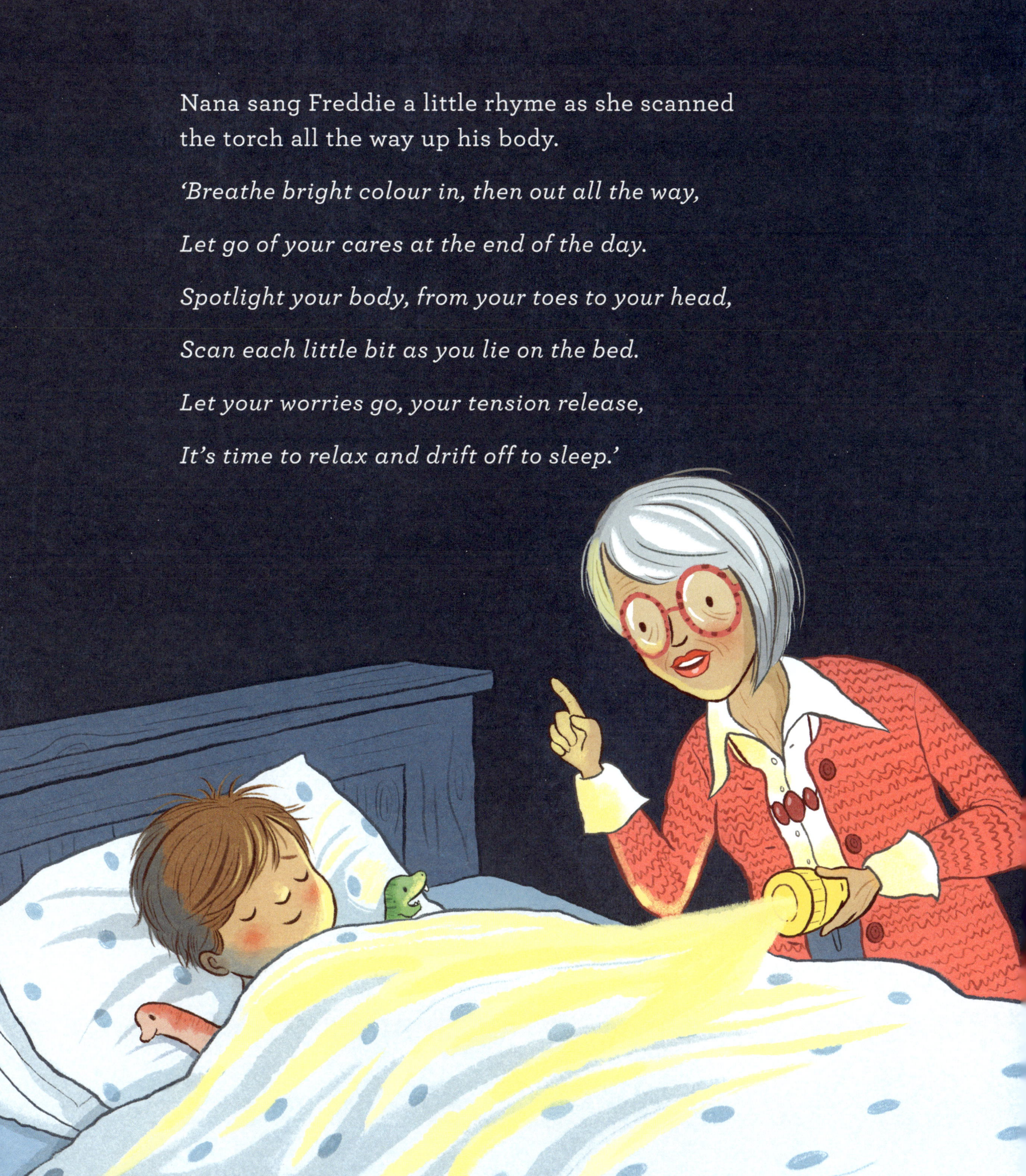

Nana sang Freddie a little rhyme as she scanned the torch all the way up his body.

*'Breathe bright colour in, then out all the way,*

*Let go of your cares at the end of the day.*

*Spotlight your body, from your toes to your head,*

*Scan each little bit as you lie on the bed.*

*Let your worries go, your tension release,*

*It's time to relax and drift off to sleep.'*

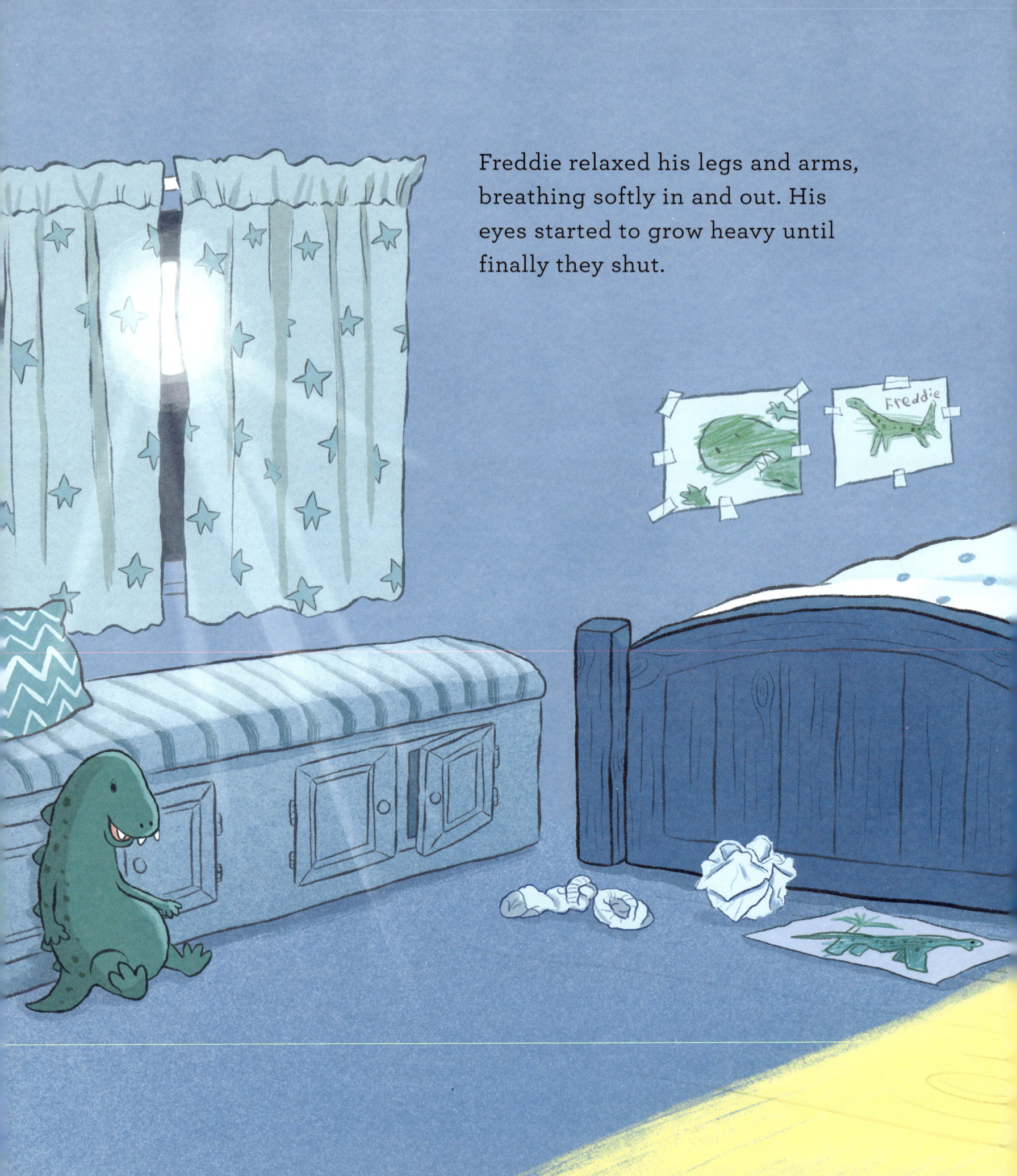

Freddie relaxed his legs and arms, breathing softly in and out. His eyes started to grow heavy until finally they shut.

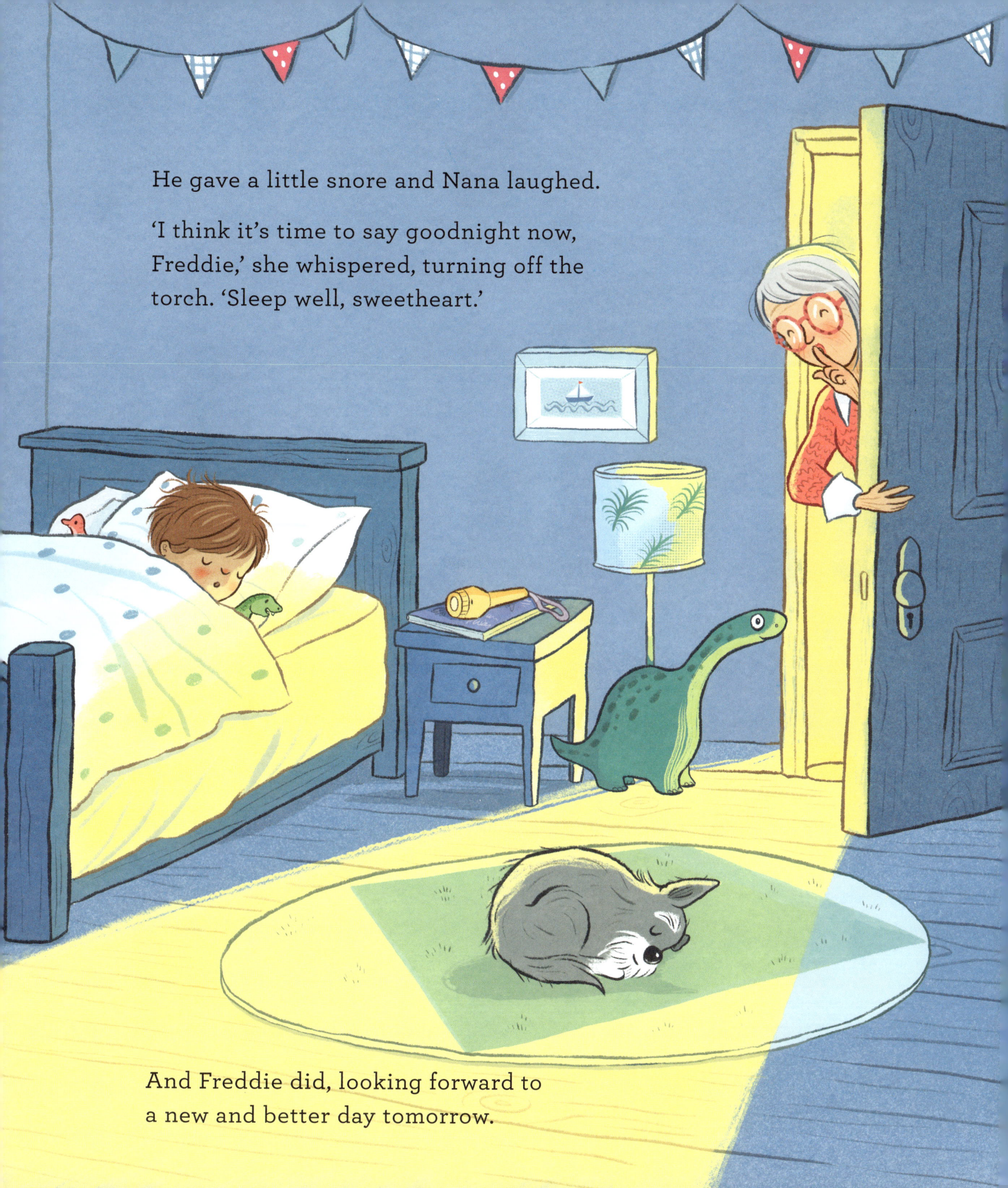

He gave a little snore and Nana laughed.

'I think it's time to say goodnight now, Freddie,' she whispered, turning off the torch. 'Sleep well, sweetheart.'

And Freddie did, looking forward to a new and better day tomorrow.

We've all had nights when we just can't get to sleep,
or when we've tossed and turned the whole time –
and it can make the next day much more difficult!
Nana's sleep scan is a great tool to help you calm
down and drift off to sleep.

Why don't you give it a try?

•

# THE SLEEP SCAN

Breathe bright colour in, then out all the way,

Let go of your cares at the end of the day.

Spotlight your body, from your toes to your head,

Scan each little bit as you lie on the bed.

Let your worries go, your tension release,

It's time to relax and drift off to sleep.

•